LIVING LABORATORIES

Women and Reproductive Technologies

ROBYN ROWLAND

LIVING LABORATORIES

WOMEN AND REPRODUCTIVE TECHNOLOGIES

INDIANA UNIVERSITY PRESS
Bloomington and Indianapolis

The paper used in this publication meets the minimum requirements of American National Standard for Information Sciences–Permanence of Paper for Printed Library Materials, ANSI Z39.48-1984.

Manufactured in the United States of America

∞™

Library of Congress Cataloging-in-Publication Data

Rowland, Robyn.
Living laboratories : women and reproductive technologies / Robyn Rowland.
p. cm.
Includes bibliographical references.
ISBN 0-253-34999-0. – ISBN 0-253-20760-6 (pbk.)
1. Human reproductive technology–Moral and ethical aspects.
2. Human reproductive technology–Political aspects. I. Title.
RG133.5.R685 1992
176–dc20 92-13199

1 2 3 4 5 96 95 94 93 92

For the Rainbow Lorikeet

CONTENTS

ACKNOWLEDGEMENTS

In the ten years since I began work in this field, a great deal has changed in the human capacity to interfere with procreation. In 1984 when I coined the term 'living laboratories', I was concerned about *in vitro* fertilisation—now the term has a fuller meaning explored in the following pages. In the struggle to understand what science is doing and to develop an analysis of it *as* it occurs, I have been partnered by many women who have inspired and collaborated with me. Renate Klein has given me a friendship based in powerful collaborative work, a partnership without competition which once again makes a lie of the myth that women can't work together. Christine Ewing has been both friend and confidante and has brought to my analysis a scientific challenge which has informed my position. For their love and friendship I will always be grateful.

The women in the Feminist International Network of Resistance to Reproductive and Genetic Engineering (FINRRAGE) have been a constant source of support: in particular Sarah Ferber and Lariane Fonseca. Three of the women with whom I founded FINRRAGE have been crucial in the development of my work: Gena Corea, Janice Raymond and Jalna Hanmer. Their friendship, their sharp insights and the debates we have had have buoyed me up when the powers of science and capital seemed overwhelming. Many others have assisted in this book in the sending of newspaper clippings and scientific articles. Some women cannot be named because they work in jobs where their political positions cannot be made publicly known. I thank you all.

Tim Curnow and Teresa Pitt sustained me with their constant faith in my work over a considerable period of time! Judy Barber, Judy Waldie, Bev Bartlett and Jan Wapling in the Deakin office typed papers relating to this book, and their arguments and discussions surrounding the work have inspired me with the belief that this information can be made accessible to all, and have helped to sharpen my arguments. Janice Maljers and Julie Melican helped compile footnotes and check references, but more importantly have given me the nurturing of friends in difficult times.

The writing of this book has taken six years and in the last three Margaret Anderson has typed and retyped until she knows every word by heart! My thanks to her for her patience and diligence, and for the excellent job she did with a fully dictated book which was then totally restructured and cut in half! Once again Sarah Brenan did the pruning, and a better editor is not to be had. She helps make the words strike clear and straight.

My mother Gwen, before she died prematurely in 1990, was a constant source of newspaper clippings and arguments. Her courage, intelligence and sensitivity taught me much. Her love and support, and her increasing understanding of the outrageous devaluing of motherhood, made me see that there is a truth worth fighting for. It was a privilege to support and nurture her in her dying.

My father Norm has always inspired me with his sense of community duty, his unstinting devotion to housing for the aged, and his ability to weigh the pros and cons of an argument. His continuing faith in the possibility of a just world and his abhorrence of violence towards others has been a sustaining part of my own value system. His love is part of my daily strength.

Finally, I thank Nigel Wood for his love and partnership. We met over our outrage against IVF Australia and continue to share a commitment to social change, a belief in a future that is not in the control of dehumanising forces, and a political activism that changes its form but not its intent with the years. He has listened to the ranting and raving, the reasoned argument, and the pain I felt when political campaigns became personal and the rumours and innuendo hurt. Though our lives are difficult to organise, the constancy of his being part of mine and I of his is the solid foundation I treasure.

LIVING LABORATORIES

Women and Reproductive Technologies

INTRODUCTION

REPRODUCTIVE CONSCIOUSNESS: THE LOSS OF INNOCENCE

Imagine women coming to maturity in the next century—less than a decade away.

> These will be women who, from their earliest days, grew up with IVF, embryo transfer, surrogate motherhood, artificial wombs, and sex predetermination technologies. They will be women who have never known a world without 'superovulation' and 'ovum capture'. From childhood, these women will have watched television news reports involving the 'Storage Authority', that is, the board in charge of frozen sperm, eggs and human embryos.
>
> They will be women whose own 'mothers' may have supplied the egg from which they were generated, *or* the uterus in which they were gestated, or perhaps neither. These women of 2050 will know that among women, there are egg donors and there are breeders or gestators and there are those who provide various body parts and fluids used in reproduction (for example, urine from which hormones are extracted for use in superovulating the ovaries of younger females). But no one woman

> procreates a baby all by herself. This will be so because by 2050, use of the new reproductive technologies will have expanded beyond the original category of women—the infertile—for whom it was first touted.
>
> This, then, might be the reproductive consciousness of our daughters in the 21st century: 'Reproduction is a complicated intellectual and technical feat performed by teams of highly skilled men who use, as raw material for their achievements, the body parts of a variety of interchangeable females'.[1]

This vision of our future may seem shocking, yet it is certainly feasible. When talking to high-school students about reproductive technology I usually end by looking at a conversation a journalist had with Dr Brinsmead of Newcastle University in which he said: 'A fetus that is not even born could ultimately have children'. He explained that immature eggs could be harvested from a female fetus at its fourteenth week, brought to maturity, mixed with sperm, and used to create a child.[2] At the moment, students respond to this with disgust, calling it 'repulsive', 'horrifying' and 'unnatural'. They are shocked and revolted, just as their parents would have been merely ten years ago if they knew that by the 1990s there would be storage banks of frozen human embryos in most major countries of the world. Yet the same students readily accept the existence of these banks and the fact that sexual intercourse is not the only way of having children. Already their sense of how humans are created is vastly different from that of their parents—just as ours is different from our parents'. We have all been affected by the softening-up processes which mould our reproductive consciousness, reshaping our sense of how people are and should be created. Few people in the 1990s blink when they hear the words 'test-tube babies', and terms like 'in vitro fertilisation' (IVF) and 'cloning' are commonly used even though it is less than two decades since the first IVF baby was born in England.

Yet despite the continuing development of the new reproductive technologies, people remain basically in the dark about how they work and about the continuing research which pushes so-called benign technologies into the more bizarre areas like Brinsmead's concept of the 'fetal mother'. They are not aware of the high failure rates and costs of the technologies both to individuals and society. The social effects are masked because the technologies are presented as a solution to individual problems. Subtly, step by step, we are changing the nature of being human and eroding the control which women have had over procreation. In its place, male-controlled technological intervention is beginning to determine how children will be conceived, what kind of children will be born, and who is worthy of receiving these new products of our science.

CHANGING SOCIAL VALUES: COMMODIFICATION AND CONTROL

There is a common belief that ideas or theories are somehow separate entities inhabiting a place called academia, remote from reality. So the scientific control of reproductive technology is often debated as if it is an intellectual exercise, while in the laboratory and in the market place increasing scientific control over procreation continues. At the same time we accept an increasing commodification of all things. Education, knowledge, information are now 'products' to be bought and sold, along with the new 'products of conception'—which used to be called 'children'. Even the 'self' is packaged and marketed in courses on how to 'sell yourself'. The ideology of family is used to sell reproductive technology, with babies up front as the sales pitch. Babies sell products; babies become products.

One newspaper account exemplifies this when discussing so-called 'surrogate' mothers:

> Its first product is due for delivery today. Twelve others are on the way and an additional 20 have been ordered. The 'company' is Surrogate Mothering Ltd and the 'product' is babies.[3]

The precedent for this has been the packaging and selling of woman as object. Advertising uses women's bodies and sexual availability this way, and an entire industry of pornography reaps its profit from this objectification. With the new reproductive technologies women are further objectified and fragmented, dismembered into ovaries and eggs for exchange and wombs for rent. The commodity 'woman' or a part of woman can be used to produce the commodity 'child'. And the product had better be perfect. As Herbert Krimmel wrote, 'It is human nature, that when one pays money, one expects value'.[4]

The product will be 'man-made' (*sic*) and therefore better than nature; and because our society does not accept the imperfect, women will be placed under more and more pressure to use all technological means offered to secure perfection. Less and less assistance will go to those who make the 'mistake' of having an imperfect child. So in the age of the perfect product, difference (named 'defect' or 'abnormality') will be less and less acceptable.

Implicit in this is our increasing desire for control—control over nature, genetic problems, difference, ageing, death and fertility. Men in power, the makers of ideas and systems of control, construct a make-believe world in which 'free choice' exists, in which individuals supposedly make choices about their lives unhindered by social responsibility to others. In this view of society, the way power works is subtly hidden behind claims for personal autonomy.

Belief in human control is used in order to reduce human fear of risk. But risk—risk of being hurt, of death, of a handicapped child, of a sudden disability or illness—is in the nature of life. The 'control myth', the myth that we have choice, leads people to believe that they are free, that there is no need to challenge those in power.[5] It also places responsibility for the down-side of the world—poverty, illness, domestic violence—on the individual and not on structures of power. The illusion of freedom is a powerful control mechanism (see Chapter 8).

Though our whole society is changed by the new reproductive technologies, initially they affect women most intimately. A history can be traced of the continuing battle between the two social groups, men and women, over the control of women's fertility and procreative potential. This battle is also drawn around race and class lines, and governments constantly develop systems structured to control which women have children, when, how and how many. The new reproductive technologies extend their power to do so in ways unimaginable a few decades ago.

Mary Shelley, at the age of nineteen in the book *Frankenstein* (1816), saw the perils of this enterprise. Frankenstein, the creator of a monster, lacks the imagination to envisage the implications of this desire to control the creation of life. Thinking only of his own expected glory, he muses to himself:

> a new species... a new species would list me as its creator and source; many happy and excellent natures would owe their being to me. No father could claim the gratitude of his child so completely as I should deserve theirs.

His monstrous creation, who seeks only companionship and love, eventually destroys those loved by Frankenstein, and in the end the creator himself. In his suffering the monster cries:

> Oh earth! How often did I imprecate curses on the cause of my being! The mildness of my nature had fled, and all within me was turned to gall and bitterness.[6]

In the popular imagination, he has taken on the name of his creator, Frankenstein, conflating the scientist with the monstrous. How visionary has Shelley's work been?

CRUMBLING MOTHERHOOD: MEN AND THE CONTROL OF REPRODUCTION

Women have mothered within patriarchal structures, in societies where men as a group have made the laws, constructed and controlled ideology, run the economy and structured social frameworks such as the nuclear family to suit their own needs and to maintain their power and privilege relative to women. As Carole Pateman points out, paternity 'refers to a form of political power'.[7]

Under patriarchy, dominance and control are defined as strength; compassion is defined as weakness. There is a deification of 'objectivity', yet it is a guise for male subjectivity. Masculine definitions of power stress domination rather than empowerment, and individual decision-making is lauded over informed consensus. Objects are valued above relationship. The control of women and children becomes essential to the definition of manhood—indeed, the powerful need the powerless, to substantiate their power and their 'right' to it.

In the relationship between men and women as social groups, patriarchal values and structures effectively set the limits of women's choice. Social institutions such as the family reinforce and maintain the patriarchal system. The economic system, where women are forced to be either totally or partially economically dependent on men, also shores up masculine power, as does the legal system, which legislates women's contractual obligations to men yet fails to contract men's responsibility to women and children (see Chapter 7).

Ideologies, or belief systems, support these social structures, so that the less powerful come to believe that the relative differences in power are natural and acceptable. Men as a social group work to convince women that they are 'naturally' worth less, are 'naturally' mothers, and so must 'naturally' be responsible for domestic labour. These ideologies keep women tied into economic dependence and domestic, physical and emotional servicing of men. People develop within ideologies to which they are so accustomed that they do not question them. Some of the 'control' myths about women are: that they should be selfless and self-sacrificing; should be 'for' men in a sexual, economic and emotional way; are less able, intelligent, creative and powerful than men; and are in a position of lesser power because of a 'natural' inclination. Moreover, to be a 'good' woman, a woman really ought to be a mother.

Men limit women's power by controlling their access to resources such as money, time and physical strength, but also to other economic resources and social resources such as the law; from their position of power men can reward women by giving them access to these resources, or withdraw access as a punishment.[8] While women are constrained socially, these power plays also operate on a personal daily basis: the politics of intimacy between the sexes may include anything from the power to influence or make decisions about holiday journeys to the minutiae of non-verbal communication.[9]

In her analysis of the social contract which establishes civil society, Carole Pateman argues that the original social contract is sexual, giving men political right over women and sexual access to them. I would argue further that inherent within this sexual and social contract is the reproductive contract. Marriage is established not only to allow men sexual access but also reproductive control. Men have always been concerned with controlling women's fertility and the 'products' of that fertility. That control has ranged from laws which circumscribe women's access to contraception and abortion to religious and political controls which set the appropriate rates of reproduction for women.

Historically, there has been increasing control by men over women's reproduction. There is a history of the elimination of women healers by a rising male-dominated medical profession and the encroaching of this profession into women's control of birth.[10] That control, extending to control over pregnancy and now conception itself, has dangerous implications for women.

There are a number of reasons why men want to control women's fertility and reproduction. First, at a social and political level, people can be seen as a resource. Reproduction, Elizabeth Moen argues, is 'a political and economic act with enormous public consequences, and this is the major reason for the control of women'.[11] She outlines political motives for fertility control such as the need of minorities to increase their numbers in order to develop a stronger power base; the desire in some non-industrialised countries to increase their size to counter in some sense the power of Western capitalism; the reduction of fertility in other overpopulated countries in order to increase per capita economic benefits; and in terms of national protection a sense of strength in numbers. This kind of thinking can be seen in reverse in the current anxieties expressed by Western nations about increasing so-called Third World populations.

Second, at the individual level, in some societies, fathers have benefited materially from the labour of their children. This has been true in countries such as India, but also in Europe and the United States of America.[12] Fathers can see children as an investment for later life, and therefore a resource worth controlling. Judith Lorber has indicated that this has always been a fundamental conflict between women and men:

> Who makes decisions for whom depends on who controls scarce resources, and children are probably the most precious scarce resource. Because of the physiological and emotional centrality of the mother–child unit, the way men can gain control of the means of reproduction is to have women under their domination... Lack of intense paternal investment or not, men in our society seem to want children of their own. They must, therefore, maintain some control over the reproductive capabilities of women.[13]

Finkelstein and Clough noted Smith-Rosenberg's argument that this desire for the control of children is 'characteristic of material societies, particularly those societies where the status of the child's legitimacy has consequences upon the distribution of private property'.[14] This would apply to most Western countries where inheritance is usually through the male line and the male heir is seen as a younger representation of the father, both symbolically and physically. As children prospectively hold property rights, there is an increased necessity for men to strengthen their control over these children and therefore over the women who bear them.

Men also demand emotional servicing from women. They often lead their emotional lives vicariously through their wives. When a child comes into the relationship, because of its total dependence and vulnerability, a woman's attention and emotional giving is drawn to the child and of necessity away from the father. A struggle for the woman's attention is created between father and child, and because of this men need to exert control and authority over both mother and child.

Third, in an analysis of consciousness, the male desire for control springs from male alienation from childbirth and procreation. Psychoanalysts have written extensively on the theme of womb envy. Freud's case studies document fantasies by men and boys for women's organs and functions. Anecdotal data abound concerning boys' desires to develop breasts and to give birth.[15] Men's fascination with and envy of women's procreative ability has also been represented in myth and rituals. For example, in some societies *couvade* is the male imitation of childbirth which can include the mutilation of the penis to resemble a vagina and male imitation of the pain of childbirth to the point where the father-to-be actually takes to his bed. Myth also represents male desire to control reproduction. The Greek god Zeus gave birth to the goddess Athena by swallowing her mother and giving birth to her through his head; he also sewed Dionysus into his thigh in order to carry that pregnancy to term.

Though men initially thought the mystery of pregnancy and birth lay entirely within women's hands, once they realised they had a role by delivering the seed, they attempted to inflate this role. Early scientific anatomists actually concealed their observations that women contributed to the fetus. 'Their rationale was that as Nature had hidden from sight the sexual organs of women, so women's contribution to a new life also should be concealed.'[16] In the seventeenth and eighteenth centuries, scientists developed the belief that sperm carried within it the minuscule human being, the homunculus. The woman was merely a vessel that cared for the developing male seed.

Men and women experience reproductive consciousness differently. The fact that men provide only the seed in reproduction ensures what Mary O'Brien calls their alienation from genetic continuity.[17] Because women bear the child and labour at birth, that have had (until recently anyway) the certainty of their essential participation. As Carole Pateman has written:

> No uncertainty can exist about knowledge of maternity. A woman who gives birth is a mother, and a woman cannot help but know that she has given birth; maternity is a natural and a social fact... Unlike maternity, paternity is merely a social fact, a human invention.[18]

Men, excluded from this certainty, have tried to annul their alienation from reproduction by the 'appropriation of the child'. O'Brien sees this experience reflected in obstetrics, to which men have brought 'the sense of their own alienated parental experience of reproduction, and have translated this into the forms and languages of an "objective science".[19]'

This alienation can generate a frustration which results in 'feelings of inadequacy, jealousy or hostility toward the female'; women are immortal in a way in which men are not. Women can regenerate themselves, but men need women in order to regenerate themselves. Azizah al-Hibri argues that men remake 'the female's womb and breasts, making them his and divorcing them from their biological functions' in sexual appropriation.[20]

These theories of alienation and envy in reproductive consciousness resulting in male control and violence towards women can be explored in the elimination of midwives by male midwives in the nineteenth century. That development represented the beginning of male-dominated medical control over pregnancy and birth. Through modern reproductive technology men limit their alienation and increase their control further. They are now capable of conception itself. They can take the egg in their hands and inject the sperm into the egg through micro-injection techniques. In this sense they become symbolically both mother and father to the in-vitro-created child. A man can rent a woman's womb to carry his child for him and in what Carole Pateman describes as 'a spectacular twist of the patriarchal screw, the surrogacy contract enables a man to present his wife with the ultimate gift—a child'.[21]

Importantly, as men decrease their alienation by appropriating conception itself—taking women's eggs from their bodies—they alienate women from their own reproductive processes, changing the certainty women once had about reproduction. No woman on a reproductive technology programme can know for sure that the egg or embryo placed back inside her body was that which came from her body.

Men are also appropriating the self of woman through this process. This is most obvious in the slavery of so-called 'surrogate' motherhood. The man is not buying merely a service, but the woman herself. The service cannot be delivered unless the woman herself is delivered.

> The self of the 'surrogate' mother is at stake in a more profound sense still. The 'surrogate' mother contracts out right over the unique physiological, emotional and creative capacity of her body, that is to say of herself as a woman.[22]

Finally, the male desire for control of reproduction lies also in the nature of power itself. Being the dominant group, men expect to control all social resources, including reproduction. But women, the subordinate group, have had exclusive control over the process of pregnancy and birth. Men may deliver the seed but it is the processes of a woman's body which bring the embryo to fetal life, and then produce a live child. Men have only been able to experience that vicariously through women's discussions of it. Men cannot accept their exclusion and have constructed institutions to invade that realm of women's experience.

Supported by the ideology of the 'patriarchal family', the 'control myths' of self-sacrificing motherhood and womanhood, and male definitions of women as irrational, incompetent, defective, dangerous and an object to the male subject, men as a social group are using the vehicles of science, medicine and commerce to establish control over procreation. It is therefore within the power dynamic of the oppressed and the oppressor that men will not allow women to retain their monopoly over reproduction and birth. Discussing 'surrogacy', Pateman writes that:

> men have denied significance to women's unique bodily capacity, have appropriated it and transmuted it into masculine political genesis... thanks to the power of the creative political medium of contract, men can appropriate physical genesis too... Now motherhood has been separated from womanhood—and the separation expands patriarchal right. Here is another variant of the contradiction of slavery. A woman can be a 'surrogate' mother, only because her womanhood is deemed irrelevant and she is declared an 'individual' performing a service.[23]

Procreation and birth are a resource which women have and men want. All forms of creativity carry a certain power; in this instance, the resource of another human being is created as well as the subject of love and affection. Like all groups who 'own' a capacity such as this, women want to hold onto their exclusivity, which is part of the group identity of women. They are the group that has the potential for giving life. In a world in which not a great deal belongs to women, this has been something which does. If what was offered to women was a sharing in the joy and creativity and limited power of procreation and birth, they might view men's desire to enter the reproductive arena differently. But as it expresses itself in a destructive and woman-hating invasion of women and their bodies, it can never be welcomed.

In the process of trying to end their own alienation, men have made procreative alienation a reality for women, divorcing women from their wombs, eggs and embryos—

from their own bodily selves and their sense of procreative continuity. They have made children products of the nexus between commerce, science and medicine, calling experimentation on women and human society 'therapy' and camouflaging the intention to map and control human genetics with the rhetoric of 'helping the infertile'. In this process women have become the experimental raw material in the masculine desire to control the creation of life; patriarchy's living laboratories.

PART 1

Motherhood, Medicine and Men: Who's in Control?

1. IN VITRO FERTILISATION: MAN MAKES THE EMBRYO

The first 'test-tube baby' born was Louise Brown, who arrived in England in 1978. She was followed in 1980 by Candice Reed, born at the Royal Women's Hospital in Melbourne, though the research had been carried out jointly by this hospital and the Queen Victoria Medical Centre. The Monash University/Queen Victoria Medical Centre/ Epworth Hospital IVF team headed by Professor Carl Wood introduced a new regime into IVF: they became 'the most sophisticated test-tube group in the world by using fertility drugs'.[1] This marked the beginning of the worrying number of multiple births on IVF programmes internationally. The first test-tube twins were born in 1981 and in 1983 the first IVF triplets were born in Australia. The same year saw the first baby born through a donated egg in Australia and, in the United States, the first baby through embryo transfer from one woman to another.

Notably it was in 1984, the year Orwell made famous, that the first test-tube quads were born and the first major debate in Australia over the 'ownership' of embryos took place after the death of Elsa Rios. The Rios case was one in which a woman from outside Australia had been admitted to an IVF programme, had two attempts at IVF, left her frozen embryos in storage at Epworth Medical Centre and later died in a plane crash. It was a year before the hospital knew of the death of Mrs Rios and it opened up an enormous debate in the community concerning the fate of these embryos.

In 1985 the first baby created by sperm extraction and IVF was born to the wife of an infertile man, and the first baby from a frozen and then thawed embryo was born in Australia. In North America, the birth of the first sex-predetermined IVF baby took place: it was a boy. In Israel in 1985 two women without ovaries became pregnant using a new method of hormonal treatment, involving the use of donor eggs and IVF.

In 1986 Australia produced the first set of twins from a frozen egg, as well as a child born to a woman whose sister had donated her egg. In 1986, the first test-tube quins were delivered by caesarean section in London. The following year the first grandmother who was used as a 'surrogate', through an IVF programme in South Africa, delivered triplets for her daughter. Finally in 1988, what is thought to be the first case of 'sister surrogacy' on an IVF programme took place in Australia, when a sister became the birth mother for a baby created from her sister's egg and donor sperm. In 1988 and 1989, scientists succeeded in carrying out the act of sperm penetration itself when micro-injection enabled them to force open the shell (zona pellucida) of the egg and inject one sperm to enforce fertilisation.

This brief summary of some of the historical moments in the history of IVF indicates the rapid speed of development of the technology and the way in which IVF has been used on an increasingly broad range of women.[2]

WHAT HAPPENS IN IVF?

> I remember the first embryo transfer I had. At the time there were visiting doctors from IVF programmes around the world, and I happened to be one of the guinea pigs

> going in for the transfer on the day they were at the hospital. It was embarrassing enough lying there with your legs up in stirrups without a room full of people staring at you and with a huge spotlight (theatre light) shining on your genitals! When my doctor said to me that after that day I would have an 'international fanny' I was really annoyed at this remark, and the innuendo that I should somehow be thrilled at the prospect of being seen by all these international doctors.[3]

These words of a woman undergoing in vitro fertilisation (IVF) present a very different picture to that popularly portrayed in the media. How has this experience become part of the so-called 'treatment' for infertility?

The original procedure in IVF was one in which the egg was taken from a woman, the sperm from her husband or partner and the two were put together in fluid in a Petri dish (hence 'test-tube baby'). If an embryo resulted it was placed back inside the woman's womb to enable implantation and possibly pregnancy. It was intended to be used by women who had blocked or diseased fallopian tubes.

Though this procedure is simply described, the practical experience of IVF is more complicated. Women who have usually undergone the exhaustive procedures of infertility testing, followed by the invasive procedures of IVF, talk about the frustration and irritation of the constant testing process: blood tests, urine tests, post-coital tests, ultrasounds, and visits to hospitals late at night and early in the mornings.[4] Mazor has described the testing process as intrusive and even 'assaultive'. She writes, 'Patients must expose their bodies for testing and procedures; they must also expose the intimate details of their sex lives and their motivations for a pregnancy to their doctors'.

Investigations often include:

> for the woman, a daily temperature measure to determine whether and when she ovulates; biopsies of the uterine lining during the phases of the menstrual cycle to determine its responsiveness to hormones; introduction of gas or dye into the uterus and tubes to check for blockage; direct visual examination of the tubes with an optic instrument (laparoscope) inserted through the abdomen; blood hormone assays, immunologic and chromosome studies; cultures to detect any infections that may prevent conception.[5]

Few women who undergo infertility investigation and treatment are prepared to discuss the processes in public because of their 'sordid and humiliating nature',[6] for example, during the post-coital test. This test supposedly enables the doctor to assess whether the sperm is viable in the woman's cervical canal and whether the mucus from the woman is resisting the passage of the sperm.

> Consequently, this test dictates that patients have sexual intercourse at a time specified by their doctor and then rush to the hospital. There the woman undergoes a vaginal examination during which the fluids around her cervix are sucked out using a cannula, a sort of straw, so that they can be examined under a microscope. In contrast to the techniques of in vitro fertilisation and embryo transfer, using a straw to suck seminal fluid from a prostrate woman's vagina is most unlikely either to appear shown step by step in a television documentary or to appear on the agenda of the meetings of government committees.[7]

Repeatedly women discuss the difficulty of 'making' their husbands have sex with them before the post-coital test. Some men just cannot perform according to the doctor's timetable and some find it humiliating and will not.

> I said, I have got an appointment at 10 o'clock, we have just got to do it. He refused. We had a terrible argument. He kept saying that sex should be a thing of beauty. I just said, that's too bad, you have got to do it now. There is no time for discussion. So eventually he stormed out. He left home. I remember him stomping to the end of the road, and as he went out, he knocked over the pot plant in the hall and the cat went scurrying and the soil went everywhere. That was at about 3 o'clock in the morning. Eventually he stormed back into the house and came to bed and we had another row. I kept saying he had to do it. Eventually he calmed down and agreed. I had to use the douche and while I was in the bathroom he made a cup of tea. Finally, we made it at about 4 o'clock in the morning.[8]

Often the test does not work. So many women have to undergo this procedure over and over again, the humiliation growing with each attempt.

> I had an endless process of post-coitals which became more and more degrading. I felt nothing much at all at first, but lately it has become demeaning, just going in and opening my legs and going through all that again. The more it goes on, the more undermined I feel, and the less I want to go there each month.[9]

The information given prior to these tests often fails to convey the nature of the experience involved. For example, one of the tests to determine whether the fallopian tubes are blocked is described as one in which 'dye is injected into the uterus and information obtained through low-dose, carefully monitored X-rays'.[10] Compare this bald statement with the following description given by a woman in West Germany:

> Totally unsuspecting, during the lunch break I made my way to one of the large X-ray practices in the city. Sitting

> on a sort of gynaecological examination couch, my lower body bared, I was greeted by the radiologist. A tearing pain went through me when he injected the 'contrast meal'. After the examination, blood was flowing from my vagina. Without a word, I received an intravenous penicillin injection and a prescription for penicillin tablets, which I was to take over the following days in order to prevent any infection of the lower abdominal region. When I left the practice, wobbly at the knees, I was quite decided not to do this. Two hours later, while I myself was examining a patient [she was a doctor], I was suddenly gripped by a cramp in my lower abdomen such as I had never felt before. I spent the next few hours curled up on a couch in my boss's room. How I cycled home that evening still remains a mystery to me. I then swallowed the penicillin tablets with an air of desperation. Subsequently I learned in discussions with other women that the pain and cramps did not only occur in my case, but are typical. This X-ray examination, the result of which showed no abnormality, was the prelude to the events of the following weeks.[11]

Such stories are related over and over again. The process is described by the woman as emotionally and mentally stressful and physically exhausting. There is little wonder that they often experience extreme depression throughout infertility treatment.

SUPEROVULATION

Women may have an embryo implanted which has come from their own egg, or from a donor egg, donor sperm, or a donor embryo; but whatever the method of selection of the embryo, all women who give eggs either for themselves or for other women are superovulated by taking fertility drugs—that is, the woman's body is made to produce more than the normal one egg per cycle, in what scientists call 'egg harvesting'.

Women who go through superovulation include the woman who is on a programme because of her own fertility problems, the woman who is donating an egg to another woman who cannot produce eggs herself, and those who have been asked to donate eggs when they are undergoing a hysterectomy and in some instances have been offered a free sterilisation as an inducement. Egg donors may sometimes be relatives, as in the case of surrogacy/IVF between sisters, or donors may be anonymous, recruited through ads in the newspapers. Many of these women are healthy, fertile, and function normally. A regime of superovulation may also be used on women entering artificial insemination by donor (AID) programmes who are there because their husbands are infertile, with the assumption that the production of more than one egg might increase the chances of fertilisation.[12] 'Surrogate' mothers in the US have also been superovulated since at least 1983 in order to increase their chances of becoming pregnant.[13] Finally, the technique of micro-injection of a single sperm directly into an egg to assist infertile men requires the superovulation of their often healthy and fertile women partners to produce a 'harvest' of eggs and therefore embryos to increase the chances of successful IVF.[14]

Superovulation can lead to fifteen to forty eggs per cycle maturing, instead of the usual one. Women are given hormonal cocktails to induce this abnormal egg maturation, one of the regular ingredients being a drug called clomiphene citrate. This drug is best known as Clomid, which is marketed by Merrell Dow Pharmaceuticals, and as Serophene produced by Serono.

There is a debate in the medical literature about how clomiphene citrate actually works. Originally it was used to prevent ovulation, then it was seen to induce ovulation. In 1984 Merrell Dow indicated that 'the exact mechanism of action in humans is unknown, but it is postulated that

Clomid acts by stimulating the output of pituitary gonadotrophins'. By 1987 the description is still tentative: 'the ovulatory response to cyclic Clomid therapy appears to be mediated through intense output of pituitary gonadotrophins...'[15] The assumption is that clomiphene acts on the hypothalamus, a gland at the base of the brain which controls the pituitary gland, which in turn determines which hormones are released into the body. It seems that clomiphene is interpreted by the body as an anti-oestrogen and tricks the pituitary overriding 'mechanisms which allow for dominant follicle selection to occur', so that many eggs instead of one are ripened in the ovary.

But clomiphene alone was not producing enough eggs and sometimes did not encourage the ovary to release them once they were fully developed so it is now often used in association with other drugs. One of these is human menopausal gonadotrophin (HMG) which is a purified preparation of gonadotrophins extracted from the urine of post-menopausal women. It is often administered as Pergonal, and works directly on the ovaries. Women are also often administered a further stimulant, HCG (human chorionic gonadotrophin), often marketed as Pregnyl, to stimulate the release of the eggs. HCG also promotes implantation of the embryo, as it is the hormone produced by the developing embryo and later by the placenta. But when administered artificially, it is used to 'induce ovulation *at a precise time* [my emphasis] on IVF and related programmes'.[16]

New drugs are being developed which may be used in association with those above, such as that sold under the brand name Buserelin (Hoechst Laboratories) and Decapeptyl (Ipsen Bio-Tech). This drug actually throws women into premature menopause. Together with the drugs mentioned above, Buserelin makes it possible for scientists to control a woman's body cycles totally. One drug blocks the natural cycle, another stimulates the ovaries by working on the brain, and yet another stimulates the ovaries to mature and release eggs by acting directly on the ovary itself. One practitioner said, 'The aim of the treatment is to reimpose a normal rhythm over a disordered one, to recover a virgin soil' (*sic*).[17] It is used on 'poor responders'; that is, women who did not produce a lot of eggs when they were stimulated; and is also given to 'non-retrievers', those who only had a couple of eggs collected. Scientists indicate that Buserelin is particularly useful 'in women who prove resistant (*sic*) to other methods of treatment'.[18] It is unclear precisely how the administration of these drugs actually affects the complex reproductive system. Anne Rochon Ford quotes one American biologist as saying:

> The gynecologist/obstetrician is probably more of a medical empiricist than any other specialist; that is, the gynecologist administers hormones as a treatment because they work and not because there is a clearly-defined understanding of their action in the body.[19]

I will take up the dangers involved in using these drugs later in this chapter.

EGG 'HARVESTING'

Egg harvesting has usually been carried out via a laparoscopy. In this operation the physician

> places the woman under general anaesthesia. Then he pumps inert gas into her to distend her abdomen and provide room for him to move and work on the internal organs. He tilts her head down 20 degrees so the intestines fall back by gravity. He makes small incisions in the abdominal wall to allow the insertion of instruments among which is the laparoscope, a slender optical device. The instrument contains a bundle of quartz fibres able to transmit light in irregular paths and produce images by

means of lenses and mirrors. Light is passed from one end of the device to the other inside the woman's body.[20]

Because of the use of general anaesthetic this operation is not without its dangers. To date, two women have died in Perth due to anaesthetic problems on IVF programmes, and one woman has died in Brazil.[21] There is also the danger of puncturing other organs within the body and of excessive bleeding once the follicles are punctured and the eggs removed.

In order to overcome these dangers, and in the name of finding a cheaper and quicker way of collecting eggs and therefore increasing the patient intake, medical scientists have developed newer forms of egg (oocyte) retrieval, using an ultrasound scanner as a guide. Initially it was introduced in order to avoid the risks of general anaesthetic and to reduce costs.[22] Because it can be carried out under local anaesthetic, it is much faster than collection by laparoscopy and theoretically can be done for women as an outpatient technique.[23] Doctors claim 'it makes IVF more convenient and economical, and less stressful'.[24]

One of these newer methods of collecting the eggs is often called TUDOR (Trans Abdominal Ultrasonically Directed Oocyte Recovery). This procedure uses ultrasound, and egg collection is via a needle inserted through the bladder and into the ovary. The woman has to undergo the procedure with a 'full urinary bladder' which needs to be filled for an hour before 'scheduled pick-up time'. She is pre-medicated (made drowsy) and the size of the bladder is checked by ultrasound. 'If the bladder is too extended, the patient is asked to void a volume corresponding to the estimated over-filling. This does not seem to be a problem for these patients, who have practised bladder filling during the ultrasound monitoring of the cycle'. Sometimes her bladder is emptied and filled with a saline solution.[25]

The puncture of the needle goes through the abdomen, through the bladder, but must 'not cut the bladder wall tangentially, because this is painful and might provoke bladder bleeding'. Lenz stipulates that the woman must be warned that she cannot move during the procedure, which takes at least half an hour, otherwise the direction of the puncture may become dangerous and she will feel pain.

> Do not forget to warn the patient since you need her full co-operation to lie still... before going into the ovary it is advisable to tell the patient that she might feel a little pain and that it is very important she does not move in spite of the discomfort.[26]

The woman's body may be continually punctured until all the mature eggs are collected. She is then advised to empty her bladder, though 'for some women it is difficult because of pain, over-distension and Pethidine [the sedative], but it is seldom necessary to use a catheter'.[27] We can assume that the woman would be 'assisted' to urinate if she does not do it voluntarily.

The transvaginal method of egg collection (also ultrasound-guided) is recommended over the transabdominal by other scientists such as Dellembach and colleagues. Though some writers have emphasised that ultrasound recovery of eggs is difficult because doctors cannot grip the ovary as they do with a laparoscopy, Dellembach et al. reject this. They write:

> In fact, the transvaginal approach is most useful when the ovaries are mobile and lying free in the abdominal cavity or when they are fixed behind the uterus by adhesions. When the patient is in the lithotomy position and has a full bladder, the oversized hyperstimulated heavy polycystic ovaries fall into the cul-de-sac.[28]

They comment that this method is 'practically painless'.

Doctors indicate that 'presumptively' ultrasound-guided egg retrieval is 'safer than laparoscopy', though complications do occur.[29] In one study, the following problems occurred in women: a puncture of the bowel confirmed in two cases and suspected in seven; puncture of the iliac vein because it was confused with a follicle on four occasions; hospitalisation of one patient due to respiratory pain in the right lung and pain in the upper right abdominal region; and cystitis in two patients. Some women were given antibiotic treatment following this egg collection. The authors claim that in spite of these problems 'a very low complication rate occurred'. Problems which did occur, they attribute to 'our beginner's difficulties', which included aspiration of urine instead of follicles.[30] One death has been reported from the transabdominal method.[31]

Some doctors have expressed concern about the new methods. Dr Platt from the University of Southern California School of Medicine is quoted as saying: 'I am worried about bleeding and infection', and that although 'no major complications arising from ultrasound-guided follicle aspirations have been reported, some have occurred. A patient in the United Kingdom required seven units of blood following transvaginal oocyte aspiration'.[32] This report indicated that the procedure cannot be done as easily as laparoscopy and that it results in fewer recovered eggs. Nevertheless, doctors push ahead with the procedure, perhaps because 'lowering the cost of IVF through out-patient care makes the technology available to more self-paying patients and also accelerates its acceptance as a reimbursable service through health insurance'.[33] Indeed, the commercial development of the tools of trade for these technologies is well under way and most ultrasound companies are marketing or developing vaginal probes.

In spite of assurances that women can undergo these procedures without general anaesthetic, it is still often used because women cannot cope with the pain.[34] As one doctor told Gena Corea and Susan Ince, 'there are some layers of the body one cannot numb'.[35] Another IVF clinic director said that unlike women in England and Denmark, his American women patients would not accept the pain: 'Here the pain threshold is not quite as good'. Corea and Ince write:

> At least 20 per cent of the women undergoing TUDOR *really* have pain. (He did not tell us how he was able to distinguish these women from others.) The vast majority he said have hematuria (blood in the urine) lasting 14-16 hours. A couple had bleeding episodes requiring blood transfusions. That bothers him.

They quote Dr Goldfarb, director of a clinic in Cleveland:

> 'The ultrasound can take a long time... because you're working with shadows'. (When the procedure is done under local anesthesia, all the time the physician is 'working with shadows', inserting biopsy probes and needles in and out of the woman's bladder and ovary, the woman lies there in pain.)[36]

In her study of forty women from IVF programmes in Australia, Renate Klein indicates that whether egg collection was via laparoscopy or ultrasound-guided recovery, women still found the experience difficult and very unpleasant. She records one woman as actually getting up off the operating table and leaving the hospital, finally fed up with the pain that this 'simple' procedure entailed. Another woman wrote:

> During my third attempt Professor X said they would use a much better technique for egg recovery. I wouldn't

> need general anaesthesia and could watch what they were doing on the TV screen. So I was quite excited and looked forward to it. And then it hurt incredibly much... I winced and could not help twitching and moving my body. Professor X was very annoyed and I heard him say to a nurse 'knock her out quickly'—which she did.

More than half of the women in Klein's study said they had negative after-effects from the egg collection. For many it was severe muscular tension and feelings of nausea and dizziness. Some complained of abdominal discomfort and three ended up with septicaemia. Four contracted vaginal infections and one had thrush.[37] The 'simpler' procedures are obviously no less traumatic and painful for the women than laparoscopy.

EMBRYO IMPLANTATION

Assuming that the superovulation drugs have stimulated enough follicles; assuming that doctors have been successful in sucking the eggs from the woman's ovary; assuming that some of these eggs become embryos; and assuming that the woman can withstand the continuing cycle of medical invasion, embryo implantation is the next stage.

Earlier methods of implantation involved placing embryos into a woman's womb, in association with ultrasound.[38] But controversies over the development of embryos outside the body, a decision by the Catholic Church that it was immoral, and the high rates of miscarriage, led scientists to develop other methods of implantation. Pronuclear stage transfer (PROST) is one method of delivery where 'the pronuclear oocyte' (i.e. newly fertilised egg) is delivered into the fallopian tubes.[39] Gamete intrafallopian transfer (GIFT) is a similar procedure, but in this case the egg and the sperm, separated by a bubble of air, are placed into the woman's fallopian tube. Both these procedures are intended for women whose husbands have a sperm motility problem;

that is, they are designed 'for a different target population than that for in vitro fertilisation'.[40]

Whether it be PROST or GIFT, the fertilised egg or egg and sperm are placed into a woman's fallopian tube using one of two methods, either through a laparoscopy, where an incision is made just under the navel, or through a laparotomy, where the surgical incision is made in the abdomen. The ethical advantage of GIFT is that the sperm and the eggs theoretically will fertilise in the fallopian tube which of course is more like the natural procedure.

A further variation on the theme involves placing of sperm into the fallopian tube.[41] This procedure, called transuterotubal implantation (TUTI) is again intended to assist male infertility.[42] In what seems to be an even simpler version of this, washed sperm are injected directly into the uterus which has been pre-programmed to ovulate with Pergonal. This technique is labelled Super Ovulation Uterine Capacitation Enhancement (SOURCE). It is 'based on the assumption that normal fallopian tubes in infertile women can capture gametes normally, said Dr Moore, of the University of Washington School of Medicine, Seattle' (apparently astonished!).[43] Dr David Meldrum of the School of Medicine at the University of California commented that 'it is becoming clear that the gametes do better in the fallopian tube than in the lab'.[44] Amazing.

And finally, in conforming as closely as they can to official Catholic teaching of fertilisation, McLaughlin and his colleagues at the Catholic St Elizabeth Medical Center in Ohio developed TOT, Tubal Ovum Transfer, which could really be called 'Man-Made Intercourse'. After superovulation the eggs are collected from the woman, then sperm is collected from a man. The eggs are then placed into the woman's tubes, while the sperm are placed in the cervix and a cervical cap is fitted to stop them escaping.

So what are the problems with these technologies? Basically there is a high risk of ectopic pregnancy, that is, pregnancy in the fallopian tube, which can lead to infertility and be life-threatening for women. As the GIFT procedure is relatively new, it is difficult to ascertain from the literature whether it is any more or less successful than IVF, but in Australia in 1988, the ectopic pregnancy rate in IVF was 6.3 per cent (an increase over previous years) and in GIFT was 4.5 per cent, both high.

But perhaps the most important point is that no matter how simple they seem, all these procedures include super-ovulation of the woman, and drug administration continues after insemination. For example, in one report of the seemingly simple procedure of TOT, intramuscular progesterone was administered from day 4 to day 25 after the procedure and HCG was given intramuscularly every other day from day 11 to day 25. In addition, progesterone vaginal suppositories were used twice a day from day 25 until the end of the first trimester.[45]

In many of the other procedures, women are given constant hormonal treatment throughout their pregnancy and often large doses of antibiotics. The procedures also continue to be personally invasive on a couple's life. For example, for one patient receiving TOT, the couple was instructed to have intercourse twenty-four hours after HCG administration and again six hours later when the ejaculation was collected in a sheath (perforated to overcome the Church's objections) and delivered to the doctors.

OTHER PROCEDURES IN THE IVF BATTERY

Freezing of embryos and eggs

Assuming that the woman has managed to remain within the programme to this point, and assuming that the technology is 'working', embryos will have been implanted, or frozen. The freezing technique allows for peculiar manipulations of family formation, as in a British case where a woman gave birth to what were referred to as 'twins', daughters born eighteen months apart from eggs collected at the same 'harvest'.[46]

Work has also proceeded on the development of techniques for freezing eggs, supposedly to avoid the ethical dilemmas over embryo creation.[47] It is presented as a 'new choice' for women. This assumes, wrongly (see Chapter 2), that the only arguments against embryo creation are based on the problem of 'when life begins'. Yet the basic and first question to be asked should be, 'where do the eggs come from?' They come from superovulated women (see Chapter 2).

The development of egg freezing has become another competitive race, made difficult by the fact that the egg is the largest cell in the body and the ice crystal formation during freezing can rupture its delicate membranes. Scientists in Britain, Melbourne and Adelaide have been working on it and in July 1986 the Adelaide team led by Dr Christopher Chen announced the first birth of twins born from a frozen egg. His new technique was hailed 'as superior in cost and chances of success'.[48] Interestingly, the woman involved had damaged fallopian tubes and wanted a child as soon as possible. She did not *need* the delay of having her egg frozen. It was a purely experimental procedure on her gametes. Chen only froze the eggs for two to three hours before thawing.[49]

Other clinics have been attempting the procedure. In a survey of 100 fertility centres internationally, Dr Andre Van Steirteghem of Brussels found that embryo freezing was performed at twenty-three centres, though egg freezing was only carried out in two by 1987. Of 228 frozen and thawed eggs, seventy were suitable for fertilisation and thirty-three were actually fertilised and replaced in a woman's body. These resulted in two abortions and only three births.[50]

In 1988 Pappert reported that clinics in Toronto were beginning the freezing of eggs and were ready to begin thawing and fertilising them.[51] In 1990, Australian and New Zealand statistics for frozen eggs indicated no pregnancies or births.[52] As a government assessment of IVF in Australia concluded, 'the results of transfer of thawed embryos have been poor; and for donor eggs very few successes have been reported. This area is clearly experimental'.[53]

What are the implications of egg freezing? Dr Chen reportedly rejected the term 'experimental procedure' when applied to this process. Instead, he called it a 'demonstrated success'.[54] The statistics do not support this claim. Researchers claim that they have introduced this technology because freezing the spare eggs created through superovulation saves the woman from having to undergo a further laparoscopy: they are doing this 'for women'. But already scientists are imagining other ways in which this technology can be used. There are discussions of the development of egg banks, similar to sperm banks. Chen, having moved to Singapore in 1987, began to talk about the establishment of the world's first egg bank. He felt it would be useful because they could be used by 'young women who wanted to store their eggs for use in later years, as well as those who had to undergo cancer treatment or had to have their ovaries removed'.[55] It is said that these eggs could be fertilised and reimplanted, 'to coincide with the woman's ovulation cycle'.[56] They could also be used to make post-menopausal women pregnant. But evidence so far of the way the medical profession works with women's 'natural cycles' indicates that women would be hormonally controlled before receiving the thawed and fertilised egg. Control would be in the hands of medical scientists who would determine which eggs were to be saved and which discarded. Just as decisions are made about 'good quality' embryos, so they will be made about 'good' and 'poor' quality eggs.

This kind of differentiation is already occurring. According to Dr Richard Marrs of Cedars Sinai–UCLA Medical Center,

> embryos are graded before and after freezing and judged on such things as cell appearance and clarity, tightness of blastomeres, and rate of growth... eventually, he foresees freezing all embryos and waiting until the woman is in a more normal [*sic*] physiologic state, rather than in the cycle in which ovulation is chemically induced.[57]

Dr John Kerin, who moved from Australia to work with Dr Marrs, said there are numerous advantages from the storage of eggs. He raises the possibility of women storing their eggs if they are faced with ovarian disease and suggests that pre-menopausal women might want to store their eggs and use them later in life. Further, he notes that eggs could be stored for women, 'when there is a temporary male [fertility] problem';[58] in other words, women's eggs would be stored 'for men', not 'for women'.

The concept of egg freezing also opens up an enormous new market which has nothing to do with infertility at all. As with the storing of frozen embryos, women would be charged for the storage of their eggs. And they could not ever be sure that the eggs returned to them were the ones that were taken from them.

Surrogate embryo transfer

A further procedure carried out in association with IVF has been surrogate embryo transfer, often referred to as 'lavage', 'conceptus transfer', or, innocently, 'ovum transfer'.[59] I prefer to use the term 'flushing', as this is a more accurate description of the process as women experience it. In this technique a fertile donor woman is inseminated with the sperm of an infertile woman's partner. She conceives and the embryo is flushed from her body and placed into the infertile woman—if all goes well.

This procedure began in the United States in 1984. Twenty-nine artificial inseminations of donor women using sperm from the husbands of the infertile women resulted in twelve embryos. These twelve were transferred to infertile women, yielding two successful pregnancies and an ectopic pregnancy, 'which was surgically removed thirty days after the transfer'.[60] One donor woman had a 'retained pregnancy' (i.e. the flushing procedure was not successful) that spontaneously aborted. (The risks to the donor are considerable. She may experience pelvic infection and/or ectopic pregnancy, 'either one of which could terminate her physiological reproductive career'.[61])

This technique was created by Richard and Randolph Seed in association with Doctors Buster, Marshal and colleagues at the University of California Medical Center, but it has been developed by a commercial company run by the Seeds called Fertility and Genetics Research. The company intends to develop a chain of clinics where flushing can be carried out. Comments by the president of the company make it clear that it is hoping to mop up the market left by the high failure rates of IVF. He told Lasker and Borg:

> If a couple can afford it and they have their own sperm and eggs, we presume they would prefer IVF. But perhaps they can no longer afford IVF or they failed [*sic*] at IVF a couple of times. Perhaps the patient can't tolerate surgery and anaesthesia anymore, whether she can't physically or psychologically. Then ovum transfer becomes a method for them.[62]

In 1981 the first donors were selected for the programme. The newspaper advertisement read: 'Help an infertile woman have a baby. Fertile women ages 20–35 willing to donate an egg. Similar to artificial insemination. No surgery required. Reasonable compensation'.[63] Since that time, couples entering the programme have been encouraged to help develop the pool of donors and they are given priority on the waiting list if they bring a relative into the pool. This puts enormous pressure on the couples and their families.

But what happens to the so-called 'donor' woman? It is not the simple procedure outlined in the advertisement. For example, it is intended that the donors will be superovulated. This is what has been done in animals using flushing. Indeed the researchers responsible for the application of this technique wrote that 'donor fecundity needs to be improved'. In 1984, Walters in the *Journal of the American Medical Association* wrote about the 'potential risks of uterine lavage—and, in the future, of possible superovulation—to the embryo donor'.[64]

Because of the potential problems of an ectopic pregnancy or a retained pregnancy, donors will be given hormones in the form of a 'morning after' pill. Women who still 'suffer an ectopic pregnancy may receive an experimental chemotherapeutic drug to dissolve the embryo'.[65] Dr Bustillo, co-director of an IVF programme at the Genetics and IVF Institute in Fairfax, Virginia, indicated that the success rate of what she referred to as conceptus transfer could be improved even further through hyperstimulation of the donor's ovaries.[66] A clearer example of experimentation on women would be hard to find.

The American doctors intend to set up centres around the country with a central computer in order to establish their donor bank. 'In a few collection centers around the country, "professional" donors will have numerous embryos washed out of them every month. These embryos can be frozen and shipped out to the OT [ovum transfer] Centers elsewhere in the country to waiting couples and their physicians'.[67] The woman is a living, breathing egg machine.

The hidden agenda has been to gain even further control over women's embryos. Buster sees this procedure as useful for pre-natal diagnosis. He has described the embryo as 'a little microchip' with an incredible amount of information in need of discovery. Buster says:

> In another five years infertility will be a non-issue, when there is an abundance of human ova available. Women are going to be much more concerned about the quality of life than they are about whether or not they can have babies.[68]

He claims that with developments in the detection of genetic diseases, and even tendencies to diabetes, heart disease and other disorders, embryos will be able to be repaired before implantation.

Keen to corner the market and make money, the company Fertility and Genetics Research applied for a patent both on the instruments used in the procedure and on the process itself. This would enable it to restrict evaluation and use of it by other researchers. The company also entered into a franchising arrangement with a group of doctors and a hospital in California. By 1987 130 transfers had been carried out, resulting in thirteen pregnancies and eight live births, according to the marketing manager.[69]

Flushing continues to be carried out internationally, in spite of its high failure rates. For example, in Italy in 1987 eight pregnancies were reported from fifty-six attempts at flushings. Donors and recipients had been synchronised in their cycles using hormones. Only four pregnancies resulted in normal births.[70] In Australia, as a result of public controversy a moratorium was placed on the flushing technique in 1984 by the National Health and Medical Research Council,[71] and so Australian researchers have concentrated on egg donation. In 1989 the Royal Women's Hospital in Melbourne put out a public call for women to donate eggs. They would need to be superovulated, but the harvesting was a 'simple procedure'.[72]

Micro-injection of sperm

In their search for an ever-expanding market for reproductive technology programmes scientists have been looking at the large population of infertile men (those with low sperm counts, or sperm which are not viable) and seeking new ways of 'helping' them. One possibility is to move women off artificial insemination by donor programmes, where husbands do not end up as the genetic and biological father, into IVF programmes where men have a greater chance of having their own genetic offspring.

In 1987, Trounson and colleagues from Monash University published a paper on the fertilisation of human eggs by micro-injection, a process in which a single sperm is injected into an egg. They argued that existing Victorian law preventing tests on the resulting embryo to check for chromosomal abnormalities should be changed:

> To ensure that the arbitrary selection of single spermatozoa for fertilisation does not result in increased embryonic abnormality, we believe that embryos arising from micromanipulation should be assessed for their chromosomal normality before the technique is recommended for clinical use.[73]

Yet researchers went ahead and implanted these untested embryos into women, literally using them as living laboratories.[74] The law was only concerned with embryo experimentation, not experimentation on women; and scientists were determined to challenge even these legal impediments. Meanwhile scientists at another hospital in Melbourne, the Royal Women's Hospital, had been using a similar technique since the beginning of 1988. This technique, called zona opening, involves making a hole in the egg's outer shell, the zona pellucida, and allowing the sperm to swim around the egg and to make an entrance. In a coy fashion, reproductive scientist Ian Johnston said: 'The difference is that with the other technique a choice is made as to the sperm. Here *nature makes the choice*' (my emphasis).[75]

'Co-culture' and intra-vaginal culture

In a procedure called 'co-culture' doctors place fertilised eggs into an 'artificial womb' created by growing the inner lining of a woman's womb in a laboratory. 'The fertilised embryos were grown in an artificial fallopian tube for two days' before being transferred into a woman. Describing the embryos as 'excellent and viable' Professor Bongso from Singapore, where the research/therapy is being conducted, said that 'they are of much better quality than that obtained in routine IVF laboratories'.[76]

In the development of an intra-vaginal culture and embryo transfer method, one to four eggs are deposited in a tube filled with a culture medium after their extraction from the woman. This tube is hermetically sealed and placed in the woman's vagina. It is held in place there by a diaphragm for 44–50 hours. It is then extracted and 'suitable embryos' are replaced in the uterus. Dr Claude Ranoux from Paris has indicated that of 100 of his patients who underwent this procedure, twenty became pregnant and fifteen delivered babies, including two sets of twins.[77]

Scientists manage to make it seem as if this has been developed for women's greater good. 'The new technique also has psychological benefits to the mother. It enables her to participate actively [*sic*] in the early stages of embryo development'.[78] So scientists try to take over from Nature, turning the woman into a 'flesh-covered test-tube'.[79]

Into her body are placed the eggs harvested through 'man-made ovulation'. Extracted by the hands of medical scientists, fertilised through either the injection of one sperm or the manipulation of many, the embryo, now a character in its own right, is placed in a test tube, and placed in an incubator—the woman.

WHAT ARE THE COSTS?

The cost of IVF to individual couples is considerable; but so too is the cost to the Australian community through government funding of health services. A report from the Commonwealth government estimates the total cost of IVF alone in 1987 as $30 million. The estimated cost to patients in this was $6 million, the government paid $17 million, while insurance funds picked up the remaining $7 million. The report estimates that the average cost of each live baby was about $40 500, with a cost to the government of $22 680. Cost per IVF treatment cycle was around $3700, of which the government contributed nearly $2700. In 1991, the annual cost of IVF and related services was about $35 million, and the government (i.e. the taxpayer) was paying 75 per cent of this (an increase on the 55 per cent in 1987). But this ignores the costs of all the previous infertility treatment, the obstetrics and perinatal costs; for example, about 27 per cent of births are premature and 34 per cent are multiple births (1979–1988 figures) and these involve expensive hospitalisation and neo-natal care.[80]

As indicated above, treatment before eggs are even collected is considerable. It involves the superovulation of women, hormone monitoring, ultrasound, and often hospitalisation. In her detailed analysis of the costs of IVF, Ditta Bartels has estimated that the total cost pre-laparoscopy to each couple is about $2700, of which the government pays almost $2000.[81] Many women have to give up their jobs and therefore their income because they cannot cope with the stress of the programme and a full-time position.[82]. Some couples travel long distances and need to stay in hotels close to hospital facilities for the period of treatment, so the financial cost to an individual couple could be far above the $6000 or $7000 mark indicated by total figures for pre-laparoscopy and pregnancy.

Although some of the costs to patients are not legitimately part of the Medicare (government) rebate, Bartels points out that accounting devices can be used to change the billing for procedures which do not have a Medicare number to procedures which do have such a number. This relabelling of services means a greater government payment than would otherwise be the case. In addition, patients often make a tax-deductible 'donation' to the research programme instead of paying for laboratory procedures, which means that they can recoup a significant part of their expenses through the taxation system.[83]

In addition, research grants from government are extensive. The funding of medical research from the National Health and Medical Research Council for 1988 indicates the priorities of scientific funding. The sum of $1 840 913 was allocated to genetically related research. IVF-related research received $433 659, while no money was given to the prevention of infertility. In comparison, community health research was allocated $160 805, cervical cancer received a total of only $232 131 and the greatest killer of women, breast cancer, received a mere $42 923. From 1979 to 1987 the NH & MRC provided funding of approximately $1 260 000 for IVF research.[84]

It is important to note that even the Australian federal government's report on IVF points out that half the units included in their study undertook research, yet:

> There was no indication that clinical research was separated from service capabilities in any of the units—in other words no patient was designated a research patient for whom no charge was raised.[85]

Women therefore pay for the privilege of being experimental subjects. As Bartels points out, because of this interrelationship between a hospital and research centre, 'the costs involved of setting up and maintaining a particular program are largely untraceable'.[86]

How much should the community be forced to pay for such an experimental (and as we will see, unsuccessful) procedure? There is a limited health budget and we could question this expenditure on such a failed scientific enterprise when in Australia Aboriginal children are dying from something as simple as diarrhoea because they do not get adequate health care. The Australian government report notes:

> IVF is a new procedure, involving new technology. It is high-cost and discretionary. In addition there are questions about the success of the procedure, the long-term safety of some drugs used in IVF and the high rate of congenital malformations and low-birthweight infants among IVF children. Under other circumstances, a new procedure such as this would be subject to assessment and evaluation before such high levels of Commonwealth funds were committed.[87]

This assessment has not taken place because scientists shroud their experimental work in the language of therapy, because they give the public a vision of IVF as happy bouncing babies given to sad infertile couples, and because the experimentation which takes place is carried out on women. Any comparable experimentation on men would not be tenable, let alone funded to such an extent.

THE FAILURE OF IVF TECHNOLOGY

The 'success' rates of this costly in vitro fertilisation process have been inflated by the medical profession so it can tout for business. Debate in Australia has raged over the rates for live births, with doctors consistently claiming higher rates than their critics. In a 1985 survey by Gena Corea and Susan Ince, to which half of the 108 clinics established in America responded, results indicated that patients were receiving misleading statistics. Many clinics were quoting a 20 per cent success rate, using what they saw as the worldwide average; yet of the fifty-four clinics which responded to the questionnaire, half had never sent a client home with a baby. 'Those zero success clinics have been in business from one month to three years and have treated over 600 women and collected, by conservative estimates, over $2.5 million in patient fees'. Statistics were manipulated, so that some of the so-called pregnancies were in fact just chemical changes which might or might not have been an early sign of pregnancy. Hospitals would cite pregnancies as a success rate, as opposed to live births, and many hospitals counted their twins and triplets in the reported totals of live births. Ectopic pregnancies were also rated in the 'success' category.[88] Most clinics use pregnancy rates because these are much higher than the live birth rates due to the high rates of ectopic pregnancies, stillbirths and spontaneous abortions. The American Fertility Society in 1988 still published its 'success' rates in terms of clinical pregnancies.[89] Similar misleading information was given to Canadian clients on IVF programmes,[90] and in Australia also, figures are constantly given in terms of pregnancies rather than the 'take-home baby' rate, though it is clear that 'from the point of view of public policy a live birth is the appropriate definition of success'.[91]

The manipulation of statistics was severely criticised by American Dr Soules in an editorial in the journal *Fertility and Sterility*. In 'The In Vitro Fertilisation Pregnancy Rate: Let's Be Honest With One Another', he wrote, 'the truth with regard to the expected pregnancy rate after IVF procedures has been widely abused (primarily by IVF practitioners... [as] a marketing ploy', and that it is competition which is encouraging this, as 'many IVF programmes in this country are struggling to treat a sufficient patient volume to maintain the programme'.[92]

Since 1984 the National Perinatal Statistics Unit (NPSU) in Australia has been keeping records on IVF and GIFT, although some units do not give all the information requested. There is some indication that this situation may improve. Fiona Stanley says that 'it is apparently now a requirement that all Australian IVF units submit their results... in order to gain accreditation by the Fertility Society of Australia and to be eligible to obtain hormonal drugs from the Commonwealth',[93] so the compliance rate may increase. The federal government inquiry also stipulated that adequate records should be kept. However, in NPSU analyses data from all clinics are lumped together. This is true of figures collected in the US and Britain also. The 'closed-ranks' attitude of the medical profession has contributed to this, preventing informed decision-making on the part of clients and real competition. If they knew the failure rates for each individual clinic, clients would obviously choose those clinics with high success rates.

It is also difficult to ascertain how many women *begin* fertility treatment. Data have not been collected on the number of women who first begin the process of IVF by undergoing hormonal stimulation. Bartels estimates that in Australia 10 000–12 000 women per year begin treatment.[94] Statistics from Diagnosis Pty Ltd indicate the dropout rates at various stages for each unit. For example, at the Infertility

Medical Centre at Epworth Hospital in Melbourne where the Monash University team works, 15 per cent of women dropped out at the egg collection stage and 31 per cent at the embryo transfer stage. At the Flinders Medical Centre in Adelaide, the statistics were 25 per cent and 50 per cent respectively.[95] In the US, Chris Anne Raymond notes that for every 100 women entering programmes for screening, less than half remain after ovarian stimulation and egg recovery, and before a transfer is attempted.[96]

Scientists continue to misrepresent their technology as effective by using the term 'success' rates. I prefer to indicate the more accurate *failure rates* of these procedures. Statistics from Australia in 1988 (published in 1990) indicate that of the over 9000 treatment cycles commenced, about 8000 resulted in egg retrieval (86 per cent) and only 776 viable pregnancies resulted (8.5 per cent), a failure rate of around 92 per cent. For every 100 women who enter a programme for one IVF attempt, ninety to ninety-five will go home without a baby. Between 1979 and 1988 only 69 per cent of pregnancies resulted in live births. Among the other women, 6.3 per cent had ectopic pregnancies and 22.6 per cent had spontaneous abortions.

There was a continuing high rate of multiple births (24 per cent), and a 'high incidence of pre-term births', and therefore a high rate of low-birthweight babies. The caesarean rate was 43.1 per cent in total for 1988, compared to the 15 to 18 per cent in the general population. The major malformation rate in babies from IVF was 2.2 per cent and for GIFT was 3.1 per cent. The NPSU report, which includes the first *reported* maternal death, concludes that 'as reported previously, ectopic pregnancy, spontaneous abortion, multiple pregnancy, pre-term delivery, low birthweight and caesarean birth rates were all more common in IVF and GIFT pregnancies than in natural conceptions'.[97] The Commonwealth government report estimated that in

1986 because of the high proportion of premature and multiple births the unproblematic live birth rate is actuallly about 4.8 per cent.

In England the failure rates are comparable, with the ratio of live births per treatment cycle averaging 8.5 per cent. *The Lancet* indicates that smaller centres may have a live birth rate of only 3 per cent and some have a total failure rate—no births at all. There is again a high rate of multiple births, with the expected rate for triplets 100 times that in the general public.[98] Figures in the United States and Canada are similar. The report from the Office of Technology Assessment in the US in 1988 indicated that initial stimulation cycles resulted in live births 6 per cent of the time. Of the 3055 clients seen in 1986, only 311 had live births, a 90 per cent failure rate.[99] In Canada, Ann Pappert reports that for the individual hospitals surveyed in her record, the most optimistic birth rate varied between 3 and 11 per cent compared with the success rate quoted in the hospitals of between 20 and 30 per cent.[100]

These failure rates can be compared with pregnancies in women who are classified as infertile and who do not use any technologies. In a study in Canada in 1983, an analysis was done of a two- to seven-year follow-up of 1145 'infertile' couples to determine whether pregnancy occurred independent of fertility treatment. Astonishingly, pregnancy occurred in 35 per cent of couples who were not treated. In addition, 31 per cent of the pregnancies in treated couples occurred more than three months after their last medical treatment, so could have been independent of that treatment. When these are taken into account, up to 61 per cent of all pregnancies occurred for couples who were 'treatment-independent'. In fact, then, such couples may be better off. The authors conclude that 'the potential for a spontaneous cure for infertility is high'.[101]

A similar conclusion was reached in an Israeli study which showed that spontaneous pregnancy in a group with a diagnosed male infertility problem occurs in 10–15 per cent of couples; the incidence of 'spontaneous pregnancy' in women with a 'mechanical factor' and one fallopian tube was 30 per cent.[102] A 1988 study of 274 women undergoing IVF in Ohio found similar results. Eleven and a half per cent of women achieved pregnancies without treatment and a further 14 per cent became pregnant after leaving treatment. As Gomel concludes: 'I think maybe we are using in vitro fertilisation too quickly without looking at...other possibilities'.[103]

Dr Marchbanks, an epidemiologist at the Center for Disease Control in Atlanta, found that of 1200 couples classified as infertile on the basis of two years of intercourse without contraception, pregnancy was later achieved in 73 per cent of cases. Of 1800 women who had failed to conceive after a year of intercourse without contraception, 84 per cent became pregnant. Although doctors use the yardstick of a year of intercourse without contraception as a definition for infertility, 'most couples who fit that standard will go on to conceive'.[104] Medical scientists may be intervening far too early in the process of conception.

These findings do not give a rosy picture of a successful technology. In fact, in any other technological area it would be considered a gross failure and immediately discontinued. Considering the expenditure and the dangers to women, these techniques should be abandoned. One Canadian clinic has come to this decision. The Queen Elizabeth Hospital in Montreal shut its IVF clinic in 1987 because since it opened in 1983, although it had had pregnancies, it had achieved no births. Dr Peter Cook, a former co-director of the clinic, is quoted as saying:

> When you say to a couple who are just scraping by and want a kid and you present them with a bill for drugs for $1000 and other charges for the medical procedure and you consider the low success rate, well, we finally said there has to come a time that enough is enough.

He said that he and his colleagues had asked themselves 'would I want my daughter or wife to undergo this procedure?': 'given the reality, the answer was no', he said.[105]

THE DANGERS

Given the high failure rates and the risks of stillbirths and birth defects, IVF technology, far from seeming a vision of science perfecting women's reproductive processes, begins to seem like a potential nightmare. And what of the dangers involved in the IVF procedures? They range from the risks associated with laparoscopy, ultrasound, multiple births, and the even more ominous potential problems from the hormone regimes used, to possible death on IVF programmes—dangers faced by women only.

DRUG-RELATED PROBLEMS

As indicated above, in superovulation a number of drugs are used in women, often in what French gynaecologist Dr Anne Cabau calls an 'explosive cocktail'. As a case study, I want to look at problems associated with one of these drugs, clomiphene citrate, bearing in mind that the inter-relationship between this and the other drugs given appears not to have been explored in detail within the medical literature to date.[106]

Clomiphene citrate is part of conventional infertility treatment. As a cocktail with other drugs it was also administered in 1988 to 86.5 and 88 per cent of Australian IVF and GIFT clients respectively, a substantial increase on the 58 per cent of women administered it from 1979 to 1985.[107]

No women were reported as receiving only clomiphene citrate.

Scientists seem uncertain about whether clomiphene citrate acts as an oestrogen or an anti-oestrogen or both.[108] Concern has been expressed about the structural similarities between clomiphene and diethylstilbestrol (DES).[109] DES was a drug administered internationally to between four and six million pregnant women from the 1940s to the early 1970s to supposedly stop miscarriage.[110] Some of the women who were given this drug were used as experimental subjects and were told that they were taking a vitamin tablet. There was a time-bomb effect with DES, and years later two to four million daughters of these mothers are now suffering cancers of the vagina and cervix at a rate higher than that of the female population of their own age. They also experience increased rates of infertility, spontaneous abortions and ectopic pregnancies. Sterility problems have also been detected in some sons of DES mothers. More than thirty years after they had used the drug, the women who took DES are also suffering from 40 to 50 per cent higher rates of breast cancer than other women of their age.[111] Notably, in spite of these proven adverse effects, the drug continues to be sold in so-called Third World countries.[112]

In a study by Gerald Cunha in California, the differences and similarities between DES, clomiphene and tamoxifen (another anti-oestrogen used to treat breast cancer) were studied in the developing human female genital tract. Though the doses administered were large, the researchers found that 'clomiphene and tamoxifen elicit changes in the human fetal vagina comparable with those of DES'.[113]

Scientific literature on clomiphene citrate is disturbing. Some studies noted the development of tumours in animals and others found that ovaries would atrophy in dogs and rats.[114] But more disturbing are the studies of children born after clomiphene-induced pregnancies, and reported cases of illness and death in women taking the drug. The *Mims Annual* (the doctors' official drug handbook) indicates that of fifty-eight children from 2369 pregnancies to mothers who were treated with clomiphene, four were stillborn, fourteen were in multiple pregnancies and among the remaining were abnormalities such as Down's syndrome (five), congenital heart lesions (eight), microcephaly (two) and a variety of other problems. Eight of the fifty-eight children born were to mothers who had inadvertently taken clomiphene during the first six weeks after conception.[115]

Cases of ovarian enlargement in both the mother and child have been reported, as have neural tube defects and vision problems.[116] Anencephaly (children born with only a brain stem) is also a concern. In 1973 Dyson and Kohler noted that 'drugs that stimulate ovulation have not been included in the list of possible or probable aetiological factors of anencephaly; the only abnormality with which they have been associated is multiple pregnancy'.[117] In a further study in 1978, researchers recorded two further cases and noted other sporadic case reports of anencephaly occurring after clomiphene.[118]

Studies in Japanese, Swedish and Australian hospitals indicate that the rates of abnormality in children born after clomiphene treatment are around 2.3 per cent compared to a 1.5 to 1.7 per cent occurrence in the general population.[119] Researchers do not necessarily conclude that there is a connection with clomiphene citrate from these studies. Yet the research on chromosomal abnormalities of egg cells after clomiphene administration suggests a link may be possible. A cluster of such studies has drawn attention to the possible detrimental effects of clomiphene on developing egg cells. In France, Sweden, Germany, and Canada, studies indicate a high rate of chromosomal anomalies and this may be one of the elements which accounts for the low success rate of implantation of embryos resulting from clomiphene stimulation.[120]

Even though researchers continue to find what they think to be birth defects and chromosomal anomalies in eggs after clomiphene use, they persist in suggesting that more studies need to be carried out before the drug can be seriously questioned. An example of this is a study by Lunenfeld in Israel. His approach is:

> There has been no evidence that the daughters of women who took clomiphene during pregnancy are at risk of reproductive difficulties, but relatively few such women have reached adulthood since the drug became available, and conclusions must be delayed until an extensive post-pubertal survey can be performed.[121]

The procedure envisaged by the medical profession seems to be to continue administering clomiphene citrate until the numbers of acknowledged long-term anomalies reach 'statistically significant' proportions. This attitude of 'wait and see' means that women and their daughters are maintained as experimental test sites for drug regimes.

Instead of the drug being seen as the potential problem, women themselves are blamed, particularly older women who show 'ageing of the ovum'.[122] Asked to comment on the disturbing statistic on birth defects on Australian IVF programmes, Dr John Yovich, at that time president of the Fertility Society of Australia and head of an IVF programme in Perth, said that the problem could arise with laboratory techniques, but that '*it was more likely to be a factor in the women themselves*' (my emphasis).[123]

Part of the problem with the birth defects rate may be related to the possibility of the long lifespan of clomiphene. If the drug is still present in a woman's body while the embryo/fetus develops, damage could be done, for example, to the developing reproductive tract. Clomid may affect a woman's body after she stops taking the drug:

> Although there is no evidence of a 'carry over effect' of Clomid, persistent spontaneous ovulatory menses have been noted after Clomid therapy in some patients.[124]

A number of studies have expressed similar concern.[125] Cunha and his colleagues write:

> Because of the long half-life of clomiphene in the patient, particularly those given large doses during the first half of the cycle, residues may not be cleared soon enough to prevent untoward effects on the developing fetus conceived as a result of prior 'anti-oestrogen therapy'.[126]

Most of the studies conducted on clomiphene are concerned with the children but some of the effects on women are well known and acknowledged: the possibility of multiple births and of hyperstimulation of the ovaries and/or the production of cysts.[127] The formation of cysts in a normally functioning healthy woman, who might be on IVF because of her male partner's infertility, can in turn lead to infertility in her. Ann Pappert reports a case from Canada where superovulation treatment on an IVF programme led to a burst cyst (one of three) which permanently blocked the woman's one functioning fallopian tube, thus rendering her physiologically infertile.[128]

An article in the *Medical Journal of Australia* indicates other potential problems: the body's defence mechanism against superovulation is overridden, and there may be maternal risks associated with ovarian hyperstimulation, such as thrombosis. The higher rate of multiple births causes concern, as does an unexpected low pregnancy rate and a higher incidence of ectopic pregnancies:[129] 'superovulation is not a simple multiplication of a normal ovulation'.[130]

At the Fifth World Congress on In Vitro Fertilisation and Embryo Transfer in 1987, US specialist Dr Karow discussed the case of a thirty-three-year-old woman who had developed ovarian hyperstimulation; he then suggested that yet a further drug, Danazol, should be used to counteract the effect of the superovulants.[131] Little discussion has taken place so far on the effects of *this* drug. But here again the general trend continues: the introduction of a new drug to solve problems with the administration of the old, instead of rethinking the whole concept of administering drugs which can cause women serious health risks.

A further health hazard may be cancer. No link has been proven between cancer and clomiphene but there have been some reported cases of severe and rapidly growing cancer in women after the administration of clomiphene. In one report from Queensland, Bolton discusses two cases where women took clomiphene for infertility. One woman who was twenty-eight years old had to abort the fetus after three months and lost both breasts due to cancer. Five years after being administered the drug, she died from cancer. In a second case, a twenty-nine-year-old woman had two children a couple of years apart after being treated with clomiphene. She lost her right breast five years after the administration of the drug.[132] A case reported from Bristol in England also indicated rapidly growing cancer in a woman on an IVF programme who had been administered the 'cocktail'. She developed multiple cysts in both ovaries and a tumour was found to fill the pelvis. The cancer involved both ovaries and the tumour covered the uterus and bladder. Loops of the small bowel and the appendix adhered to the mass. After massive surgery (a sub-total hysterectomy), bilateral salpingo-oophorectomy and chemotherapy, at the point of writing the paper the authors commented the woman was said to 'remain well'! They conclude that 'although hormones may not directly initiate tumour formation, they can act as promoters in the process of carcinogenesis'. They then review further studies that suggest 'that elevated gonadotropin levels are implicated in the development of ovarian tumours'. One hypothesis is that the 'incessant ovulation increases the risk of cancer by not allowing the ovary to have non-ovulatory rest periods'. A number of other researchers also express this anxiety.[133]

Professor Eylard Hall has indicated his concern that there may be 'a possible increased risk of ovarian carcinoma after repeated hyperstimulation of the ovaries combined with multiple follicle punctures', though he points out that these suppositions are of a hypothetical nature. His argument is that 'as there is some epidemiological evidence that the use of oral contraceptives reduces the risk of ovarian cancer, it might be that the disease is in some way related to the occurrence of ovulation', and that there is a need to follow closely women who have been given these drugs.[134]

In general the evidence and reports that suggest that there may be damage from clomiphene citrate are worrying. A number of papers about its nature and functioning appeared in the late 1960s and discussions about birth defects, particularly anencephaly, appeared in the early 1970s. From the late 1970s onwards, there appears to be an increase in the number of papers pointing to the promotion of cancer in the women who were given hormone therapy. Studies in the 1980s focus attention on similarities between DES and clomiphene, and intimate serious concern about long-term effects in the women who take the drug and in their children.[135]

Apart from these studies there is an astonishing array of possible negative effects from Clomid. It seems that these become more frequent and severe the higher the dose and the longer the course.

> The more common side effects are hot flushes, abdominal discomfort (distension, bloating, pain or soreness), ovarian enlargement and visual blurring...other less frequently reported symptoms include nausea or vomiting, increased nervous tension, depression, fatigue, dizziness and light-headedness, insomnia, headaches, breast soreness, heavier menses, intermenstrual spotting, weight gain, urticaria and allergic dermatitis, increased urinary frequency and moderate reversible hair loss.[136]

In 1987 were added abdominal symptoms related to 'ovarian enlargement';

> Rare instances of massive ovarian enlargement and rupture of the lutein cyst with haemoperitoneum have been reported. Visual symptoms, described usually as 'blurring' or spots and flashes (scintillating scotomata), increase in incidence with increasing total dose and disappear within a few days or weeks after Clomid is discontinued.[137]

Patients 'should be advised' that there may be the possibility of visual symptoms and that administration of the drug should stop should this occur because 'the significance of these symptoms is not yet understood'.[138]

The term 'side effects' is a weak description for such a debilitating adverse reaction as ruptured cysts which necessitate emergency surgery and potential serious health hazards such as interference with 'cholesterol synthesis' after prolonged use.[139]

It is important to note that these symptoms may come from use of the drugs with dosages indicated by the pharmaceutical companies. But superovulation, which was introduced by the Monash research team and is now used internationally, means the administration of higher doses of the drug for much longer periods of time. Though 100 mg/day is suggested as the highest dose for a period of five days, and it is suggested that this be given for no longer than three cycles, research studies indicate that higher doses are given for longer periods of time.[140] In Klein's Australian study some of the women took clomiphene for six and nine months respectively with varying dosages. I know of one woman who said she was on clomiphene for eight years. A woman in Holland was administered 50 mg per day for a five-day period, then put on 100 mg per day. After she had taken this dosage for six months, her gynaecologist put her on to 150 mg per day. This introduced terrible side effects and the regimen was changed so that 'I had to take one tablet on the first day of treatment, two tablets the second day, up to five tablets a day' (one tablet equals 50 mg). Her doctor told her that 'Clomid was an absolutely safe medicine', yet she had very unpleasant side effects:

> I couldn't deny the side effects any more. I had dizzy spells, a constant pain in the left side of my belly and a funny feeling inside my head...I couldn't see sharply any more. I saw lights and colours and I felt kind of strange/funny inside my head. I remember one time at school when I began to panic because I couldn't see clearly. It made me feel unbalanced and insecure. While working with pupils I suddenly couldn't remember the simplest things. Was that a side effect of the drug as well? I almost couldn't believe it. I also suffered from a pain in my belly which dragged on and on. Emotionally I wasn't stable any more.[141]

Research scientists obviously introduce a great deal of 'flexibility' into their administration of these drugs and their trials on women subjects, and the women are ill-informed of the potential dangers. Doctors constantly reassure their women patients that there are no side effects to these drugs.

As Dr David Healy of the Medical Research Centre at Prince Henry's Hospital in Melbourne wrote:

> Clomid is not a hormone. It is a medicine which has been used safely for more than 20 years for the treatment of infertility, which is specifically related to non-ovulation ... the side effects which the Dutch and Geelong women claimed were due to treatment by Clomid such as depression, lethargy and impaired vision are NOT consistent with the side effects doctors would expect during or after the use of this drug ... in fact the side effects of Clomid are only minimal and are no more than hot flushes or mild sweats ... the structure is NOT almost identical to DES. Medical practitioners and pharmacists are well aware of this scientific fact ... lastly, there is no evidence that superovulation increases the risk of ovarian cancer. Indeed, women who have had children have less risk of ovarian cancer than childless women. Quite simply, helping infertile women have children decreases, not increases their risk of ovarian cancer ... it is concerning and unacceptable that these scientific errors continue to appear in print.[142]

It is indeed. If doctors have this attitude to the 'scientific' facts and potential dangers of clomiphene citrate, how much do they tell their women patients? When one Geelong woman told her doctor that she felt 'depressed, spaced out, lethargic and over-emotional' the gynaecologist said this was an unusual response.[143]

In Klein's study of forty Australian women who had left an IVF programme, nine reported developing ovarian cysts. Other women developed enlargement of the ovaries, ovarian abscess and septicaemia and some reported constant bleeding. Dizziness, nausea and feeling 'very ill' are so-called 'side effects' women on these drugs report with almost no exceptions. Visual problems often occur too.

A woman in England whose initial dose of clomiphene was doubled reports:

> By this time I had discovered that my eyes were being affected. I had gone to the optician worried about my eyesight and was asked if I was on any drugs. He told me that the drug could have six possible side effects on the eye alone.[144]

For some of the women, these adverse effects do not stop when they abandon IVF. One woman told Klein: 'I have had two operations, the first was a hysterectomy, the second the removal of a cyst on the remaining ovary'. Another woman reported that she had felt depressed, emotional, unable to cope, lethargic and tired for weeks after she left the IVF programme. She wrote:

> Bloated stomach, irritated, continued to superovulate for at least two or three months afterwards. Premenstrual tension effects tripled. The worst was the continual DIZZINESS—began on the second day of the injections and only gradually improved. Even now, three months later, I still feel dizzy if I overdo things. For the first two months it was terrible. Three months after my first attempt I bled for three weeks and was very ill as I developed a severe bronchitis at the same time. Now I have a rash—three months after my second attempt. The bleeding episode in June last year was very unusual for me—my GP said it was probably connected to the IVF treatment.

An example of the 'doctors know best' attitude was expressed by the US fertility expert, Georgiana Jaciello, who calls findings on chromosomal abnormalities in eggs after clomiphene therapy 'worrisome', then goes on to say:

> It would seem prudent to view such studies of human oocyte chromosome complements with extreme caution

> in order to avoid sending a message of alarm about abnormalities that might occur in progeny after in vitro fertilisation or other treatments.[145]

So doctors seem concerned that this information might make women reconsider undergoing infertility 'treatment'. As one woman in an Australian study by Burton said:

> The Professor tells us that according to the labels and his books they don't have side effects. Once someone comes out and is brave enough to say you get side effects, other women will say so too. I think that is what he is worried about—that side effects are catching.[146]

In Klein's study, nine of the forty women were given some indication that there might be multiple births and dizziness, but that was the limit of the information given out. A woman from Holland speaks for many women when she says:

> I hadn't heard of Clomid before in my life. One of my girlfriends, a nurse, warned me. She explained that hormone-drugs could be dangerous. At that time I didn't know what to do with her words. I desperately wanted to believe the gynaecologist. *He was the authority and I thought he would know best* [emphasis added].[147]

Women should be wary of putting such trust in medical 'experts' who refuse to inform them of the possible dangers involved. The suspicion that this is not unintentional is reinforced by a recent French medical text:

> IVF is a remarkable instrument for testing new ovulation procedures thanks to: the parameters it allows to be controlled; the number of women who can be treated. Lastly it enables controlled series to be carried out which compare the new therapeutics with 'routine' stimulation protocols. It no longer appears possible to consider the

> marketing of new drugs for stimulating the gonadic-pituitary axis unless they have been tested within the framework of IVF.[148]

Drug companies like Serono, the sole supplier of Pergonal in America, have sales which in 1986 reached $35 million.[149] Does this kind of profit motivate doctors and pharmaceutical companies to take the 'wait and see' approach which seems to be advocated in the medical literature? If so, the victims of this 'experimental methodology' of trial and error will be the women who are taking the drug and, potentially, their children.

It is worth bearing in mind the reasons for the use of these superovulation procedures. A paper by Zorn, Boyer, and Guichard indicates that it is very inconvenient to have women ovulating during the weekend. Titled 'Never On A Sunday: Programming For IVF-ET and GIFT', they gave their patients injection after injection in order to develop what they called a 'flare-up protocol' to control the moment of ovulation, commenting that 'any method that avoids the need for clinical and laboratory staff to be on duty seven days a week should be considered, provided the results are not impaired'.[150] Other doctors write of IVF and egg recovery as outpatient procedures, pointing out that by the use of 'menstrual postponement followed by a fixed protocol of stimulation' the working week for doctors can be restricted to five days. They suggest enlisting self-help groups and counselling in order to gain acceptance of these procedures:

> Support and information are not only important for the couples in reducing stress but also help to *ensure compliance* [my emphasis] with the complicated procedures required for in vitro fertilisation.[151]

In perhaps the most gross irony, the daughters of women exposed to DES who are suffering from infertility due to physical abnormalities, who have repeated ectopic pregnancies, or who are unable to carry a child to term, are being encouraged to join IVF programmes. In one study, these women were superovulated using the hormonal cocktails.[152] As Anne Rochon Ford writes:

> In our lifetime, we have seen birth deformities from thalidomide, vaginal cancer from DES and infertility from the Dalkon Shield IUD. How many more discoveries like these will it take before the parties involved—the pharmaceutical industry, doctors and patients—realise that they are part of a continuum?[153]

Part of the new regime of superovulation may involve the use of other drugs such as Buserelin in order to throw the woman into premature menopause before controlling her cycle.[154] Though analysis of this drug has yet to be completed, Françoise Laborie has already sounded the warning. She obtained from the manufacturers of the drug a brief report (with no references) on animal research; different doses had been given to seventy-five female rabbits and forty-five rats, and studies showed that although the rabbit fetuses developed normally, rat fetuses showed retarded development. The conclusion by the manufacturer was that *'no malformation was observed'* (my emphasis).

Before producing menopause artificially, Buserelin creates a 'flare-up' which can produce hyperstimulation and cysts on the ovaries. One French doctor working near Paris noted at the Fifth International Meeting of IVF Researchers in Norfolk, USA, in 1987 that two women out of seven previously treated with Buserelin had severe problems. One was hospitalised for several days and another developed enormous cysts which had to be removed. In addition, an Australian woman has given a personal account of how close to death she came after hyperstimulation on Buserelin. Four months after treatment she had developed advanced breast cancer, though a mammogram before IVF treatment had shown no such indication. She links her cancer with the Buserelin and hormonal cocktail administration.[155]

Scientists are currently developing new procedures which they say may eliminate the necessity for the superovulation of women, though whether a drug-free regime will ever be possible has yet to be determined. Research is proceeding in Australia, England and the US on the maturation of immature eggs in vitro, by taking slices of women's ovaries and developing the eggs within them. In 1987 Vines reported that Ian Gordon at the University College, Dublin, was harvesting immature eggs from the ovaries of cattle carcasses and maturing them within the laboratory. He had fertilised the eggs and created embryos. Also working in this area was Christopher Polge from Animal Biotechnology, Cambridge. In 1988, it was reported that Barry Cross from the Institute of Animal Physiology and Genetics Research in Cambridge had gone a step further than Gordon in perfecting the system for obtaining the eggs.

> The Irish technique does not involve continuous in vitro culture; instead, the ova dissected out of the slaughtered cattle are fertilised in vitro, but are then grown up in the uterus of a sheep. When the fertilised ova are sufficiently mature to be ready for implantation, the sheep is slaughtered and the embryos extracted.[156]

In Australia, Dr Max Brinsmead, a reproductive physiologist at the University of Newcastle, suggests that a slice of a woman's ovary containing several hundred immature follicles could be taken. 'We could then grow the follicles to maturity and harvest the eggs as they're needed'. He claims that 'this would result in a healthier patient and more receptive uterus at the time of embryo transfer and could lead to a greater rate of successful pregnancies'.[157] (Professor David Armstrong at the University of Western Ontario has supposedly matured eggs in this way and had successful pregnancies in rats.) The development of ovum banks and the use of immature eggs was given a 'boost' by research in Korea where immature eggs were collected from surgically removed ovaries and fertilised to form embryos. Triplet girls were created from this project; the first time live children were produced. For scientists this would also overcome the egg donor shortage they face because women on IVF do not want to donate their eggs.[158]

An endless supply of eggs to experiment with would make the dream of British IVF pioneer Robert Edwards come true—he yearned over ten years ago for 'egg heaven'.

IVF PROBLEM BIRTHS

Many people may feel that multiple births are a joy to infertile couples because they wanted a family and now they have one! But they are problematic. The multiple birth rates on IVF are high (24 per cent) because up to three or four embryos are transferred into a woman. The rate of caesarean delivery rises according to the number of babies, so these rates too are high (see p. 92).

There are a number of problems with multiple births apart from those which obviously affect the woman. Congenital abnormalities occur in multiple-birth children three times as often as in the normal (non-IVF) population.[159] The public rarely hears about these problems with IVF. In probably the only newspaper report on such a case, John and Sally Bloomfield were interviewed for the *Sydney Morning Herald*. Their daughter Elizabeth was born with spina bifida; she had a gaping hole in her back and a malformed spine. She may never walk and will probably be incontinent for life.

> For little Elizabeth, the next twelve months will be one operation after another. She has already had a tube

> inserted in the back of her skull to feed spinal fluid to her brain. Next, she must have operations to rearrange the bones in her hips and knees and transfer muscle to her legs in the hope that she may be able to walk. Meanwhile, Elizabeth's legs will be encased in plaster, which is replaced each fortnight, to keep them straight.[160]

The NPSU statistics indicate that extremely low-birth-weight children are 'more common in IVF and GIFT programmes than in normal conceptions'.[161] Outcomes for these children can include blindness, severe disability, deafness, cerebral palsy and other health difficulties. In one study of sixty survivors of extremely low birthweight, at two years of age though 74 per cent had no important disability, 17 per cent had moderate disability and 9 per cent were severely disabled.[162] A further follow-up study found that despite intensive-care techniques 'they are still significantly more physically and mentally impaired than normal infants', having more hospital readmissions, more operations, various problems with physical and mental growth and a greater prevalence of cerebral palsy than normal-birthweight children. Dr Neville Newman, Director of Neonatology at the Royal Hobart Hospital, commented on this:

> The technical skills and equipment that result in the survival of VLBW infants are readily available, but this is merely the beginning of what may prove to be a long and arduous life of disability...evidence from studies of children with chronic or severe illness suggests that the pattern of family functioning may be disturbed markedly.[163]

In Britain and Australia the birth of triplets, quads and quintuplets resulting from fertility drugs and from reproductive technology programmes is beginning to cause concern because of the impact on the care then available to other children. When sextuplets were born prematurely in Cambridge in England, they effectively closed a special-care baby unit for three months. Dr Cliff Roberton said: 'From May to July we had to turn away more than thirty pre-term babies. God knows where they went. In order to have six babies we put thirty at risk'.[164]

In one case which became one of international interest, a woman in England was given Pergonal as a fertility drug and delivered sextuplets, three months prematurely, and she and her husband had to watch as one by one the babies died. The babies were being kept alive with various incubators, ventilators and drips because they could not breathe unaided, could not digest food and could not control their body temperatures.[165]

Discussing anomalies in multiple births, Hendricks writes:

> We are faced with the undeniable fact that the human species is not designed to carry more than a single fetus in utero with any degree of biologic grace. The observation that the anomaly rate among twin infants appears to be more than three times the anomaly rate in the general population is only a single indicator of the seriousness implicit in human multiple pregnancies. As long as multiple pregnancies occur in humans, twin fetuses will continue to bear a triple burden of poor growth in utero, mal-development in utero, and the threat of a high perinatal mortality.[166]

Because of the problems with multiple births, the British Voluntary Licensing Association has restricted implantation of embryos to no more than three. Professor Ian Craft refused to accept the guidelines and was not licensed for a year by the VLA, but there are no other sanctions for such non-compliance. In Australia, public concern was raised by triplet and quadruplet births in Perth. Dr John Yovich had ignored the guidelines of the Fertility Society and was implanting more than the recommended three embryos. His accreditation was taken away and he took legal action. Again, there is no effective way of enforcing the limit.

Popular media representations of multiple births are always extremely jolly, with happy smiling triplets on the front cover of women's magazines. The difficulties of carrying and delivering and caring for multiple-birth children, particularly if they have been born with problems, are stories rarely told. For most of these multiple births, post-hospital assistance for mothers is not available. In England and in Australia it is very difficult to get government-funded home help if you have triplets or twins. In one example, Hon Campbell in North London was virtually housebound for a year with her triplets.[167] In 1989, one Perth woman had to relinquish three of her quads for adoption because of the strain associated with their unwanted arrival. People looking for 'a' child do not always welcome four. Some of the children are constantly hospitalised and ultimately some are institutionalised. After the pain and grief of infertility, to go through this experience must be devastating.

I do not want to make value judgements about the quality of life experienced by people who are born disabled. Obviously the greatest problems for these children, apart from their health, are social attitudes to their disabilities in a society which stresses more and more the child as 'perfect product'. But we also need to look at the effects on women of bearing 'problem' children. (Because of men's abnegation of responsibility in child-rearing, women will be faced with most of the burden of caring for these children.) No one has assessed this aspect of IVF.

So what do scientists do about these potential problems? They do not stop using fertility drugs. They do not implant only one embryo. Instead, true to their history of limited vision, they develop a new technological trick. This is called 'reduction' of a multiple birth. In this process, using ultrasound, a needle is inserted through the woman's abdominal wall and manoeuvred into the fetus. A small dose of potassium chloride is injected into the heart of the developing fetus to 'terminate' it. The technique is carried out in the first trimester of pregnancy. Eventually the dead fetus is absorbed into the woman's body or delivered with the live child.

Many of the women on whom the procedure is used have taken fertility drugs or had four or more embryos implanted through IVF.[168] Most 'reductions' are carried out on a woman carrying more than two fetuses, and it has been reported as used on women carrying five, eight and even nine fetuses after having taken Pergonal.[169] Most reductions leave twin fetuses in the woman's body because the women have obviously undergone extensive infertility treatment of one kind or another, and hope that one at least of a set of twins will survive. Dr Mark Evans, described by NBC television as a 'selective reduction specialist', says that he leaves twins because 'we are afraid if we go down to one, there is no margin for error'.[170]

In Australia, the first recorded termination of this kind was carried out on a woman pregnant with twins. A male embryo, 'at risk of haemophilia', was selectively destroyed. This reduction was carried out at ten weeks following screening by chorionic villus sampling, a new genetic screening technique (see Chapter 2). The woman then gave birth to a healthy female child.[171] Thus, this procedure can also be used for 'reduction' on genetic grounds. As with other technologies, its uses tend to be generalised as time goes on to broader groups in society.

The risks in these procedures include spontaneous abortion of the remaining fetuses, internal bleeding and infection. The procedure is still 'a risk to the mother and to the continuing pregnancy', and bleeding in the uterus 'could cause lifelong neurological damage to the remaining infants'.[172]

Other side effects and dangers from this procedure will only become evident as it is used more widely. The experience itself must be extremely painful for the women, as for each 'reduction' the needle has to be reinserted through the abdominal wall. Again, instead of relinquishing control over the whole process, stopping the administration of fertility drugs, stopping the implantation of more than one embryo, doctors resort to even further bodily invasion of a woman in order to control 'their' pregnancies.

OTHER RISKS

As the statistics indicate, the rate of ectopic pregnancy and of stillborns is cause for concern. The grief of infertility, followed by the 'high' of being pregnant, followed by the distress and grief after the loss of a child or a potential child, increases the burden of loss for women undergoing IVF and GIFT.

There are other issues of concern too. There is an extensive use of ultrasound during fertility treatment and during pregnancy on IVF. Ultrasound is a method of bouncing high-frequency sound waves off a dense tissue mass. The reflected signals are transformed into electrical impulses and thrown onto a screen; thus doctors can actually get a visual image of the developing fetus, or of the developing follicles after superovulation drugs have been given. But the effects of ultrasound are still uncertain and have not been effectively studied. One study showed that, ironically, the use of ultrasound to check on the growth of follicles 'reduces the fertility of the patient'. The authors also noted that 'the absence of harmfulness of this diagnostic technique in ovulation has not been demonstrated'.[173]

Although ultrasound is said to be safe, 'as with other radiation, it is questionable whether there is a threshold level below which ultrasound is safe, and to what extent the effects of exposure are cumulative over time'; some say its hazardous effects are 'legion'. Although women are told not to worry about ultrasound, as Ruth Hubbard points out, 'that is also what we were told about X-rays'.[174] Dr Mendelsohn, Professor of Paediatrics, Preventive Medicine and Community Health at the University of Illinois, has criticised the use of ultrasound. He is concerned that exposure to ultrasound at the fetal stage may cause harmful effects which would not be revealed for twenty to fifty years. He notes that it has not been declared a safe method through regular testing. Mendelsohn quoted an Oxford survey which found that in 1983 five-year-old children who had been exposed to ultrasound in the womb were developing leukaemia and other cancers in higher numbers than unexposed children. After their five-year follow-up the authors concluded that full data would not be available until the children had been followed for twenty years. The evidence is not conclusive, but there have been no long-term studies which showed that the procedure is safe.[175]

An American National Institute of Health panel warned in 1984 that ultrasound should only be used when necessary and that it carried 'hypothetical risks'.[176] Tests on animals had shown that the procedure could cause retarded growth, impaired immune response and chromosomal damage. But these studies in a US laboratory were carried out on fetuses outside the body and with very high levels of ultrasound, so they are not necessarily relevant to human patients. Nevertheless in America, Britain and in Australia, the medical associations generally recommend that ultrasound should not be used routinely on pregnant women. Yet on IVF this is a regular procedure. Women may undergo many ultrasound experiences before a child is actually born, assuming they are one of the lucky ones who become pregnant.

Caesarean section is common with IVF. There is a two to five times higher risk of maternal morbidity with such deliveries. Problems with general anaesthesia account for one-fourth of deaths resulting from caesarean section (at least 75 per cent of maternal deaths are considered to be preventable).[177]

Women sometimes use donor sperm on IVF and related programmes. Concern about the transmission of various diseases through these sperm have been documented. Chlamydia, hepatitis B and pelvic inflammatory disease, which can cause infertility, can be transmitted this way,[178] as can AIDS. Four women in Australia were infected with AIDS through the use of donated semen in 1985.[179] Since this event, Australian hospitals have used only frozen semen, hoping that tests carried out before freezing would indicate whether the semen was carrying any transmittable diseases.

The problem is that none of these are failsafe methods. In addition, freezing of sperm significantly reduces the number of motile sperm and the pregnancy rate is much lower than it is with fresh sperm. In general, there is little information available on the care that may or may not be taken with sperm inseminated into women on IVF and artificial insemination programmes.[180]

The risks of IVF procedures have been brought home most starkly with the reported deaths of women in Spain, Brazil, Israel and Australia. In Israel Ailsa Eisenberg died on the operating table when she was only donating an egg. She suffered a massive haemorrhage. In Brazil, Zenaide Maria Bernardo died from respiratory failure. She was undergoing IVF because 'they [had earlier] removed my tubes without my authorisation'. It was the Brazilians' first IVF experiment on five women. The newspapers reported that 'from a scientific point of view the programme had been a success: four ova, four implanted embryos, perhaps four pregnant women'. The fifth, Zenaide, died eight days later.[181]

In Australia, two women have died on the IVF programme at the Avro Clinic, now Concept Clinic, which was housed in the King Edward Memorial Hospital in Perth. In both cases there was respiratory failure, in the second case due to 'therapeutic misadventure' according to the coroner's report. In both cases the women were undergoing a laparoscopy.[182] Two Perth women have also suffered strokes possibly caused by superovulation.

In addition, the stress of IVF programmes can be dam aging. This was brought home tragically by the murder and suicide committed by the husband of a woman who had been on an IVF programme in Melbourne. Don McDermott killed his wife, Jan, and then shot his mother-in-law before turning the gun on himself. Professor Carl Wood of the Monash team indicated that it was infertility itself rather than the IVF process which was the problem: 'it was [Mr McDermott] who maybe had trouble coming to terms with his infertility'.[183] In response, a woman who was herself a long-time unsuccessful patient on IVF wrote in a letter to the *Age* that

> the mass media presents to the public the relatively few successes and medical achievements of the IVF teams. Rarely is there discussed the enormous emotional toll and extreme depression that I, and others like me, have to contend with.

She points out that there is no grief counselling for couples and no counselling to assist them after they have left the programme when it has failed them.[184]

The assumption that they will succeed places enormous stress on women: when the programmes fail them, they experience it as a failure in themselves. Reproductive technology makes it harder for people to come to grips with their infertility. The tragic consequences mostly remain undocumented. But in the instance above, and in the deaths of other women on IVF programmes, we can see that reproductive technology is not without its lethal 'adverse reactions'.

HOW WOMEN FEEL ABOUT IVF

Media representation of women's experiences of IVF are usually restricted to the vision of glowing happiness that comes from a successful birth. In fact, some of the few children who do result have severe problems, and most women go home without a baby. So what are the experiences of this majority? The most important studies to date have been carried out by Crowe, Burton and especially Klein.[185] In 1989, Klein published a book containing first-hand accounts of women who have used conventional infertility treatment, as well as IVF, and of surrogates who have been involved in commercial contractual arrangements in the US. In a separate study Klein also used questionnaires and detailed interviews with forty Australian women who had been through IVF.

Medical science manages to convey to women that they have 'failed', inducing a kind of alienation from their own bodies: 'I felt my body was cheating me. It had let me down'.[186] Entering into an IVF programme further lowers their self-esteem:

> It's embarrassing. You leave your pride at the hospital door when you walk in and pick it up when you leave. You feel like a piece of meat in a meat-works. But if you want a baby badly enough you will do it.[187]

Women find it extremely difficult to cope with the procedures of IVF in terms of time, tension and stress. Many of them end up leaving work in order to cope with this.[188] Women in Klein's study commented constantly on this:

> Somehow I managed to juggle work, housework, taking the kid [her child from a former marriage] to school and then rushing to hospital every morning for a whole month for blood tests, urine samples and ultrasounds.

Women are contemptuous of the so-called 'counselling' they receive and feel like experimental guinea pigs.

> I was amazed at how easy it was to get on the programme. We were not offered any counselling, so I had to find help re emotional crisis myself. I felt like a Friesian cow ready to be experimented upon. I did not feel like a person after talking to Professor X. The team aren't interested in people, only in science.[189]

They are also anxious about the techniques and the drugs involved.

> I sometimes get concerned what's going to happen to us in ten to fifteen years' time. Our generation were guinea pigs for the Dalkon Shield, and now we are guinea pigs for a new form of technology. I think it is really, really important that some research is done on the long-term effects of the hormonal treatment we are getting. Even if there were an increased incidence of ovarian cancer I'm sure a lot of women would still want to be involved with the programme but it would be necessary to have increased surveillance.[190]

The attitudes of doctors and practitioners create a general feeling of rage and anger in the women, which they are unable to express because of the power dynamics involved. They want something the doctors can give, and know that if they offend them, the doctors could reject them from the programme. One woman client, a leader in a self-help group Concern in Western Australia, wrote

> We, as patients, are not in a position to comment objectively about many IVF issues. Always we are conscious of the fact that we are in the 'compromising' position. For most couples our dearest wish is to have a child so we do not publicly complain about the endless experimental procedures, the dehumanised method of treatment, the pain, cost and emotional strain that is an integral part of IVF. I have known some to complain, but only to incur the wrath of the IVF team.[191]

Again and again women are angry because they feel they know their bodies better than the doctors, who reject their suggestions, for example, about when they are ready to ovulate:

> I said 'Look, I know my body. I am feeling that I am about to ovulate...' they didn't believe me and I had the laparoscopy only hours later. When I woke up I didn't even need to ask. I knew there were no eggs—and there weren't.

Another infertile woman commented in a similar vein:

> I know my body really well. Always had very regular periods, always knew exactly when I would be ovulating. So I told them I wouldn't need a hormone injection, to release eggs (I didn't want more hormones in my body!). They ignored me and insisted on the injection. I felt angry—and powerless.

Women try to express all these feelings to both the medical practitioners and the counsellors, but counselling is usually seen by the medical staff as a procedure for indoctrination into the programme. There is no space to work through this range of feelings. As one woman said:

> I really felt caught...when we went to the initial counselling there was no space to say any of this. We

> were given the impression that it was a big privilege to be accepted—and we were—so we had to be grateful. I shut up and began three years of utter misery...[192]

Most of the women talk about lack of informed consent, and many of them had asked again and again for information which was denied them. A woman in Burton's study said:

> Honesty is the most important thing. There are a lot of things to handle and you can handle them if you have got good information. I think it is dishonest to give a success rate based on the number of positive pregnancy tests per number of women who had embryo transfers. I think we need to know how many women are treated, how many pregnancies occur, how many deliveries occur over a period of time. I think it should be given out to patients from the outset. I think a lot of women drop out of IVF because they just can't handle the hassles because they're unprepared. I think a lot of women feel cheated because it is so financially expensive and disruptive of our lives.[193]

Women experience the failure of the technology at a variety of stages along the way—when the superovulation drugs do not work, when there are no eggs to collect, when the eggs do not fertilise, when the embryos do not implant, when they spontaneously abort, when a woman has an ectopic pregnancy or stillbirth. One woman in Burton's study said, 'I spent the day scrubbing the shower recess, I just wanted to be alone. A friend had decorated the house with pink balloons and streamers when I came home from hospital. When I got my period and told my husband he busted the balloons and tore the streamers down'. Another said, 'I just wanted to sit in a corner and die'.[194] One woman in Klein's study described her feelings of failure when her eggs were not 'good' enough:

> When I was told after the third attempt that my eggs weren't good enough and that I should give up I was shocked and utterly devastated. I remained deeply depressed for more than a year and I was suicidal a lot of the time. I felt such an abysmal failure, a barren woman unable to give my husband a child and my parents their grandchild. *I had even failed technology* (emphasis added).[195]

Many women are shown their embryos through the microscope. This 'viewing' of the embryos and the eggs allows the woman to personalise that tissue into the desired child. The cruelty and manipulation inherent in this is shown in the devastating reactions when eggs do not fertilise or the embryos do not implant. One woman said: 'When you have an egg being fertilised it's like having a baby in intensive care—you're just waiting for someone to come and tell you it's died'. Women experience the failed cycle of IVF almost like a miscarriage.

> I cried and cried when I heard that the embryo transfer hadn't worked. Ever since they had allowed John and me to have a look at our embryos in the glass dish through the microscope I had really believed it. Yes, we could have our own children, there they were... and you ache and ache but then sign on again because it seems you were so close, close as never before in your life... so you had to give it another try.[196]

In Klein's study, six of the forty couples were taken to the laboratory to look at their embryos, but many other reports indicate that this is becoming a more regular practice. It helps to explain why women find it very hard to get off programmes. One woman said to Klein: 'I felt like a hamster on a wheel. I felt sick and tired and yet I couldn't get off it. I had become addicted'.[197]

Having embryos in frozen storage is another form of coercion. Women are trapped by the possibility of having another attempt, even when everything tells them that it will fail.

> You see, it's these frozen embryos... now I don't want them to be flushed down the sink, I don't want to give them for research and I don't want to give them to another woman. So what other option is there than to go back. I know it sounds sick. Here I am feeling so angry about the programme, being totally sick of it, even having my own child... and yet, you know... you just plug on, on and on... also, I must admit I feel quite maternal towards my embryos in the fridge...[198]

In addition, the enforced control of sexual intercourse is extremely invasive. Women resent the way IVF affects the sexual relationship between partners. They are encouraged to have intercourse according to various schedules, be it by temperature charts or for post-coital tests. One woman summed this up in Burton's study:

> My husband thinks I've lost interest in him. It's not that. It's just that the whole area is so painful I want to deny it exists. The other night while we were making love I thought—'This isn't something special any more between the two of us. It's something which involves all these other people'.[199]

The picture that comes through from all these discussions with women on and off IVF programmes is of a kind of suspended life where everything is timed around IVF: the job, leisure, sexuality. Feelings of pent-up rage and anger at the humiliation of the treatment, the lack of information given, the lack of sensitivity of the research staff, and the periods of failure, are constantly recurring themes. The stories are of constant waiting, and more waiting—to hear if there are more eggs, if the husband can produce the sperm, if the eggs will fertilise, if the embryos will implant.

In Klein's study, half the women felt physically ill, depressed and emotional for a considerable time after they had left the programme. Half needed and sought counselling support elsewhere. Some found that they could not get help through the self-help groups, which they felt were uncritical. One woman commented that she couldn't 'stand their adoration of the doctors and scientists... I just don't think they are the wonderful people they make them out to be'. Women are left with emptiness and feelings of failure, though some have gained new information on the workings of their bodies and a closer relationship with their husbands.[200]

Women can and do resist these programmes. In one Australian hospital alone, 2092 patients who had entered their names on the waiting list did not commence one treatment cycle.[201] Lasker and Borg, in their survey of infertile women through questionnaires and interview, found that of the women they questioned more than a third had rejected the idea of IVF because of the poor success rate. One woman they interviewed succeeded in withdrawing herself from the programme and expressed enormous relief at having done so:

> I knew that there was a point that I had to quit. There are just so many times I could allow this kind of invasion, not only into my body, but also into my psyche. I don't know how long you can hang on to the word *hopeful.* You have to come to a time when you say it's over. It was such a relief to put it behind me and get on with my life.[202]

And one woman spoke for many in Klein's study when she summed up her feelings as follows:

> After attending hospital for two and a half hours one day, and being prodded and poked all that time, blood tests, ultrasound, needles, I eventually got off the table and said 'tell the doctor he can stick this up his jumper'.[203]

A World Health Organisation report has concluded that 'there has not been adequate research on the short-term and long-term risks associated with IVF'.[204] In vitro fertilisation is a procedure which uses women's bodies as living laboratories and invades their lives and their sense of self. Healthy fertile women are often placed on programmes for their husband's infertility and end up undergoing dangerous procedures which can lead to their ill health and possibly to death. The development of new 'improved' technologies which are more invasive, such as 'reduction' to limit multiple births, and the development of egg banks open up further avenues for the abuse of women. Finally, the drag-net of in vitro fertilisation is thrown wider and wider, through, for example, 'sister surrogacy' and the micro-injection of sperm, seducing more and more women into experimental programmes that endanger women's lives and health.

2. THE MASCULINE DREAM OF QUALITY CONTROL: GENETIC ENGINEERING

> She asked: 'Do you think it will have to continue like that?' meaning testing and abortions again and again. The [Indian] woman said: 'Yes, that's what I mean... but I will do it if only my body will take it. And I am afraid that my husband will divorce me and take a new wife who will give him sons... you just don't know what I have been going through in the last seven years because all I gave birth to were girls... it would be so much easier for me with a son. My husband and his family would respect me much more.'[1]

If women are inefficient and deficient with respect to the child-bearing process, the 'product' they produce could also do with improvement. In its desire to control the outcome, masculine science is developing procedures to create 'perfect', 'unproblematic' people, through sex determination, or through elimination of genetic illness, or through the 'enhancement' of a healthy normal adult.

The dream of quality control raises questions essential to the value structure of our society. It raises issues about eugenics, social control, and about the use of women's bodies as raw materials and as experimental laboratories. Any intervention in the structure of the embryo will ultimately affect women, because it is women who will be expected to carry these embryos through to term, to deliver the resulting children, and to rear them.

SEX DETERMINATION

There are several methods for selecting the sex of children. The most obvious and well-known method is amniocentesis at about the sixteenth week of pregnancy followed by abortion. The new chorionic villus sampling (CVS) technique which is used around week 10 also detects the sex of the fetus and may be followed by abortion if the fetus is of the 'wrong' sex. (Both these techniques will be taken up in Chapter 3.) These techniques have been variously labelled as femicide, gynaecide, and as the 'previctimisation' of women.[2] Aborting fetuses because of their sex is often justified in terms of the elimination of sex-linked genetic defects. However, while over 200 genetic defects are linked to the male, most abortions on the grounds of sex eliminate female fetuses.

A further method of sex selection involves the selection of appropriate sperm. The Japanese, for example, particularly under the leadership of Rihachi Iizuka in Tokyo, have developed a centrifuge technique for separating female- from male-determining sperm (female-determining sperm are heavier, carrying as they do 3 per cent more DNA than male-determining sperm, and have a different electrical charge). The technique is claimed to be 95 per cent effective in producing girls and 85 per cent effective in producing boys.[3] Another method of sifting out male-determining sperm was developed by Ericsson, and is practised in his chain of at least forty clinics throughout the US but also in forty-six countries in Europe, Asia, and Latin America. His advertising material indicates that out of one group of 263 couples who approached him, 248 selected boys and 15 selected girls.[4]

There is also an immunological method in which the female is immunised against proteins that exist only in male cells and sperm which are Y-bearing. Hewitt comments that there are no reports of the application of this technique in humans—hardly surprising because 'obviously this technique can only preselect in favour of females'.[5]

In the search for 'quality control' of sex, or what Ursula Mittwoch describes as 'the race to be male', geneticists are becoming more excited about the possibility of screening embryos for sex.[6] The sex of a developing embryo is not determined until around the seventh week and scientists are determined to pinpoint the switch that determines this. In 1987 Dr David Page felt he had found the single gene on the Y chromosome that was the sex-determining switch, though since then his research has been debated. He called this the 'testis-determining factor' (TDF). Emphasising the drive for maleness, writers tend to treat femaleness as a negative quality—to become female, something must be missing: for example, Joyce wrote, 'If it [TDF] is absent, the fetus develops into a female'. What no one commented on was the politically interesting point that unless there is intervention the fetus will continue to develop as female—which leads to the conclusion that femaleness is 'normal' development.[7]

The use of a DNA probe for the Y chromosome was developed at the University of Edinburgh, notably by an IVF team; another case of 'therapy' and 'research' overlapping. IVF and sex determination had already been linked in 1986 when Dr Stephen Taylor in the US announced the birth of the world's first sex-determined test-tube baby—a boy—and sex determination has also been used there in surrogacy cases.[8] The Edinburgh team indicated that the test could be used to assess embryos during IVF, or to assess embryos that were collected by flushing methods. This would mean that even women pregnant through intercourse could have their embryos flushed from their bodies, checked by pre-natal diagnosis for sex-linked genetic disorders, and replaced in their bodies. The authors comment that 'diagnosis of genetic disorders at this early stage would allow selection of unaffected pre-embryos for transfer to the uterus, thus avoiding the need for abortion'.[9] A member of the team, Dr John West, said that 'it certainly wouldn't be ethical to use the method to choose the sex of a baby. But, we couldn't prevent the technique being used that way'.[10]

At about the four-cell stage, one cell can be taken away from the developing embryo, supposedly without detriment to the rest of its development. This cell can be screened using the sex DNA probe, and only those embyros of the 'correct' sex need be reimplanted. At Hammersmith Hospital in England, scientists have established this form of sexing the embryo using a DNA probe. They have transferred female embryos only to IVF clients wishing to avoid genetic diseases passed on to boys. (Because boys only inherit one X chromosome on which a faulty gene might lie, they are not protected from this gene as girls are who inherit two X chromosomes, the normal one protecting them from the genetic disease.) Two out of five women tested became pregnant with twins. Though one of the researchers commented that 'we do not think it is ethical' to use this pre-implantation diagnosis for sex determination, he points out that 'there is nothing to stop other clinics offering just such a service for choosing a baby's sex'.[11]

Of the sex determination techniques so far available, amniocentesis followed by abortion is the most widely used. In India, although amniocentesis followed by abortion for sex determination was banned in public hospitals in 1975, private clinics do not fall under this legislation. One study in Bombay indicated that of 8000 cases of abortion, 7997 were of female fetuses.[12] There is concern about the way the sex ratio balance in India has changed since 1901.

In 1901 there were 972 women per 1000 men. In 1981 there were 925 women per 1000 men. The 'deficit' in women was 9 million in 1901 and 22 million in 1981. As Ravindra, lecturer in pharmacology in Bombay, comments, 'sex determination tests do not guarantee the birth of a male child, they merely ensure multiple abortions'.[13]

Most women who undergo amniocentesis in India do not know of its use in screening for genetic problems, but are merely using it as a sex-selection technique. In their culture, the birth of a daughter brings more pain and less status, as is clearly articulated in the quotation heading this chapter.

What are the costs to women who undergo these procedures? India has the second highest rate of maternal mortality in the world and 22 per cent of this is due to abortions. Following multiple abortions the chances of later having an ectopic pregnancy (in the fallopian tube instead of the uterus) and secondary sterility from infection or haemorrhaging increase. Yet the push for quality control over the 'products' women create continues. As one doctor said:

> In developing countries like India, as the parents are concerned to limit their family to two offspring, they will have a right to quality in these two as far as can be assured. Amniocentesis provides help in this direction.

Patel comments that 'this perverse use of modern technology is encouraged and boosted by money-minded private practitioners who are out to make a woman 'a male-child-producing machine'. She points out that doctors do not charge a great deal for amniocentesis so that even working-class people can easily afford it. Costs are particularly low compared to the dowry needed to pay for a daughter on marriage. Pointing out the abuse of women that these techniques entail, she cites an example of Harkisandas Hospital, which has a considerable reputation in Bombay. It carries out sex-determination tests but does not support abortion, so women are sent to other hospitals to have the abortion done. But the hospital asks them to bring back the female fetuses after abortion to Harkisandas for the purposes of further 'research'.[14] Highlighting the hypocrisy involved in the selective use of this technology, Patel points out that after the Bhopal gas tragedy, in spite of repeated requests by women's groups and the increased numbers of babies born with birth defects, the government refused to provide amniocentesis for pregnant women at the same time that it refused to ban the test for sex-determination purposes.

The primary argument used to support this scenario of woman abuse is population control. The aim of a nett reproduction rate (NRR) of one means that a woman should only replace herself. Female children are discouraged. Population controllers argue that it is better to prevent the birth of a female than to have her growing up in neglect and oppression. 'By this logic', says Patel, 'it is better to kill the poor rather than let them suffer poverty and deprivation'.[15] Population controllers argue that they are encouraging people to develop a 'balanced' family. But Patel points out that if a woman is creating more and more sons, she will certainly not be having amniocentesis in order to get rid of a male fetus and have a daughter to balance the family.

This assumption that women are the problem and need to be systematically eliminated, and that their reproduction should be controlled, is part of the imperialist and racist nature of the so-called First World. While using the rhetoric of women's rights, advocates of population control insist on technological and medical reproductive intervention which does nothing to change the nature of power and the distribution of resources in a country such as India. The roots of the population problem do not lie with women. The problems are a lack of food and nutrition, economic inequality, a lack of sanitary medical facilities, a lack of education for women, a lack of clean drinking water, and a lack of control over the ideology which determines the definition of woman. The state of Kerala in India is the only state where the sex ratio favours women; it also has the lowest birth rate, the lowest mortality rate, and the highest female literacy rate in the country. In contrast, regions which have traditions of female infanticide and where women are uneducated have the highest birth rate.[16]

Other countries have also been affected. China, with its policy of one child per family, practises sex determination. South Korea is so concerned about the sex ratio imbalance being created that its government has launched a TV advertising campaign which is pro birth control but anti sex selection, 'depicting the ideal Korean yuppie family as being a handsome couple with one child—a baby girl'.[17]

But what of the industrialised West? In the West Midlands of England the incidence of selective abortion based on sex has also caused concern. Some doctors were so concerned that from 1 January 1987 they determined that they would not include the sex of the fetus with the laboratory report after amniocentesis.[18] In the US, sex-determination clinics are doing healthy business. Paying a minimum of $500, couples line up at these establishments. They include 'a group of minorities' only interested in having male children, primarily from Asia, India and the Middle East; more commonly, they are young couples that include a young career woman who wants to have two children, one of each sex, rather than 'end up with a big family trying to get a boy'. Sex determination in the US appears to be an increasingly lucrative field, and the number of couples interested 'appears to be growing'.[19] In Australia, once the Japanese research on sperm centrifuge was announced, Dr Iizuka was inundated with pleas from Australians seeking to have boys.[20] A study published in *Australian Doctor Weekly* indicated that following chorionic villus sampling women were aborting fetuses because of their sex, and that these were primarily female.[21]

Studies by a variety of social scientists have shown that a majority of all societies have a strong preference for male offspring. The few communities that do value women do not do so because they signify power and status but rather because they are valuable chattels or commodities within the marriage or work markets.[22]

The most obvious consequence of sex determination is in the sex ratio. This is already changing in India, as indicated above. To date, few governments have shown concern about this. The implications of it for women can only be imagined. Currently women have the numbers, yet as a social group are the most exploited, manipulated, oppressed and brutalised group in the world. What would the status of women be as a vastly outnumbered group?

Hilary Rose argues that although sex determination is an issue of concern, it will not necessarily lead to the extermination of women. She writes that it

> may be in the interests of particular men to kill women and girls and to abort female foetuses, and for patriarchal order to use terror to maintain control, but it does not follow that it is in the interests of patriarchal order to eliminate such a useful source of labour, sexual servicing, etc. A society based on the domination of a subordinate group…does not exterminate that on which it relies.[23]

Rose is assuming that patriarchy is consciously pursued, a form of conspiracy, but patriarchy is a much more complex phenomenon. It is evident not only in institutional structures and in ideology but also in the individual unconscious. Individuals can act to uphold or extend patriarchy without being aware of it, simply by expressing a preference *for* boys, rather than *against* girls.

If sex determination were readily available, the rate of first-born males would dramatically increase.[24] First-borns have been shown in general to have more advantages over later-borns and to be generally more intelligent and achievement-motivated, more successful, more independent and high in self-esteem. Medical technology would therefore be building the traditional sex role stereotypes into a biological determinism. Males would be more stereotypically masculine; and (second-born) females more stereotypically feminine.

Interestingly, in the US, 72 per cent of the 1464 respondents in a survey said they would *not* choose the sex of their children if the opportunity were available, and 49 per cent said they thought it was a bad idea. This kind of attitude does not conflict with the predictions of people choosing males if the technology were available. What many people are saying is they would prefer that the option did not become available.[25]

One British scientist has suggested the need to stop women 'breeding'. He has suggested that women's right to work would need to be curtailed and polyandry would develop as the number of women dropped. He writes that some societies 'might treat their women as queen ants, others as rewards for the most outstanding (or most determined) males'.[26]

Some argue that because most societies favour males, the girls who are born will feel specially wanted. People will easily limit family size instead of trying for a boy or a girl after two or three of the one sex. Families will be happier because there will be no disappointment at the birth of a 'wrong'-sex child. These arguments are simplistic and sexist. Rather, women will be valued for sexual and breeding purposes rather than for their intrinsic worth as people. 'When women are scarce and men are readily available', write Guttenberg and Secord, 'a protective morality develops that favours monogamy for women, limits their interaction with men, and shapes female roles in traditional domestic directions'.[27] Campbell has suggested that the masculine values of aggression and violence will increase. 'More of everything, in short, that men do, make, suffer, inflict and consume', he writes.[28]

There are health dangers to women in sex-selection procedures. Multiple abortions increase the risk of post-operative infection, haemorrhaging and adhesions, all of which can result in infertility. For pre-implantation diagnosis, embryos created in normal pregnancies would need to be flushed out and reimplanted—or pregnancies could be generated on IVF programmes to ensure easy quality control—with all the attendant problems (see Chapter 1). There are psychological implications in sex determination too. In her study of women using ultrasound and amniocentesis, Barbara Katz Rothman writes:

> It is one thing to have given birth to a son. It is another thing to be told that the fetus growing inside your body is male... males and females are culturally defined opposites. To have a male growing in a female body is to contain your own antithesis. It makes of the fetus not a continuation and extension of self, but an 'other'... the fetus who is male is other, an intruder in the female body. The more patriarchal, the more traditional the woman, the more that is true.[29]

The class implications are even more invidious. Abortion is difficult for poor women to obtain; access to sex determination may also be class-regulated in the West or imposed on the poor in developing countries. If sex determination is associated with surrogate motherhood—and it is already being used in surrogacy—more poor women who need the money may become involved in a breeding system to create the male powerholders of the next generation. Non-surrogate women in the working class will still produce girls, sex determination being costly, while the powerful will elect for male offspring.

Sex determination is founded on and reaffirms sexist notions of the value of females and males. Few people discuss the expectations which are placed on children because of sex determination. Once people start conceiving particular kinds of children, they place upon those children expectations because of their own desires. People who select a girl or a boy are doing so because they have specific aims in mind, which can include the intention of having a child with a particular temperament, a particular nature and a particular future role. These expectations reinforce stereotypical definitions of what it is to be male and female in a patriarchal world.

GENETIC MANIPULATION

EMBRYO EXPERIMENTATION

The unique characteristic of IVF for scientists is that it made the human embryo available for experimentation for the first time; science could produce material for genetic research almost on demand. But embryo experimentation has caused much more concern internationally than medical experimentation on women. Stockpiles of embryos accumulate while governments vacillate about the extent of the research which should or should not be allowed.

At a conference in Europe in 1988 Niall Tierney of the Irish Department of Health said 'identity and integrity must be protected from the single-cell stage', but Anne McClaren, head of the Mammalian Development Unit of Britain's Medical Research Council, argued that individuality begins only after fourteen days, the deadline already set by Britain's Warnock Committee on experimentation. She argued that it is at this stage that the genetic uniqueness of the embryo is determined and therefore its identity begins.[30] Similar legislation in Victoria is the site of on-going social debate.[31] Other scientists argue that experimentation should be allowed to continue until a central nervous system is developed and the fetus experiences pain. But the fact remains that internationally at least 200 000 frozen embryos are stockpiled awaiting determination on their fate. In Britain alone clinical work on embryos was being conducted in 1988 at thirty-four centres and half of these were doing ongoing research.[32]

In discussions of embryo experimentation, scientists manage to present the embryo as if it somehow falls from heaven independent of women's bodies. But the primary question for women is—where do the embryos come from? They come from eggs. And where do the eggs come from? They come from women's bodies. But the bodies of which women?

The first group of possible egg donors are women on IVF programmes. Under superovulation treatment they produce more than the normal one egg per cycle. So-called 'spare' embryos are frozen and available for implantation or experimentation. These women are in an invidious power relationship with researchers: they depend on them for a hoped-for pregnancy, and thus are more wary of arguing with researchers who suggest that experimentation on their embryos will assist other infertile women and may reduce the failure rates of IVF. Nevertheless surveys indicate that women on IVF are not totally convinced of the value of embryo research. A survey carried out by the infertility group Concern in Perth found that the donation of embryos for experimentation was not acceptable to 35 per cent of respondents and a further 25 per cent of couples were undecided.[33] A study in The Netherlands found that 59 per cent of IVF women rejected experimentation on spare embryos and a further 23 per cent were unsure.[34] In this study, fertile women were also questioned and *none* of these women believed that embryos should be used for scientific experiments.

In a study conducted in New South Wales one IVF woman said, 'I want them to do research but not on *my* embryos'. IVF client, Dr Barbara Burton, in her representations to the Australian Federal Senate Select Committee on Human Embryo Experimentation, supported embryo experimentation but said that the embryos should come from 'normally fertile couples': 'It is the sort of area where I would be unhappy for embryos in IVF programs to be used because I think they should be used for getting infertile women pregnant'.[35]

Doctors are turning more and more to another source of eggs—so-called 'donor women'. At the moment these are primarily women seeking sterilisation. In Australia Professor Carl Wood seeks eggs from women looking for sterilisation. At least three centres in Britain are currently using embryos from donated eggs, and in 1984 Patrick Steptoe was offering free sterilisation operations to women who were willing to donate their eggs to infertile patients. Mr Steptoe commented that 'I would like to build up a panel of forty women ready to donate eggs'. He was intending to use these eggs for experimentation, which included incubating an embryo in the oviduct of a pig or a rabbit for six to twelve hours.[36]

The procedure is by no means simple. For one Austrian woman, for example, it included superovulation using clomiphene citrate, injections of ovum-maturing hormones, a series of ultrasound investigations and urine tests, blood examinations, vaginal screening, and a painful flushing of her ovaries to try to loosen the eggs. The woman in this case was selling her eggs to an institute for reproductive endocrinology in Vienna. Because this was an IVF programme she assumed her eggs were being sold to the doctors concerned for use in IVF. But of course the possibilities for embryo experimentation are also available if women are now paid for their eggs. The woman concerned received no payment if no mature eggs were collected. As she said, 'The doctors pay for the product "egg"'.[37]

In Australia in 1989, two hospitals called for women egg donors in the community to 'help infertile couples have children'.[38] One of these hospitals, Royal North Shore in Sydney, is also conducting embryo experimentation.[39] In the 1990 National Perinatal Statistics Unit report, it is indicated that at least one hospital has been conducting embryo experimentation work.[40] One wonders whether the women involved know that their eggs are not being used for IVF but for experimentation.

The increasing number of embryos stored in various IVF institutions throughout the world in itself puts pressure on governments to allow embryo research. Research in turn will generate the need for a greater market of embryos and women will be encouraged more and more to donate their eggs which will be 'useless' to them after sterilisation. Scientists argue that embryo experimentation is needed in order to reduce the failure rate of IVF, to 'eliminate' genetic disorders and to improve the screening of embryos. Ultimately the only test of whether embryo experimentation and genetic interference has worked will be for women to carry manipulated embryos and fetuses to term. As Mike Rayner, an embryologist at the University of Oxford, has written: 'If the [screening] technique is to be practicable, a high proportion of screened embryos must be capable of developing into babies'.[41] This leads us into the area of genetic manipulation.

GENETIC ENGINEERING IN ANIMALS

Animal research gives us two important issues to consider. The first is the question of our abuse of the animal world; the second is whether we should be allowing research which often forms the basis of experimentation in human beings. There is no space here to detail genetic work on plants, but a few examples illuminate the extent of manipulation and the obvious commercial motivation behind this work. Australian scientists working for the Commonwealth Scientific and Industrial Research Organisation (CSIRO) have genetically engineered a protein-rich alfalfa intended to boost wool growth when eaten by sheep.[42] Disease-resistant tomatoes and strawberries are also being developed, as are crops designed to repel pests. Scientists already claim to have isolated the gene responsible for making tomatoes go mushy and are attempting to stop the softening process. Flowers too may be 'designed to order': research in Amsterdam is creating mottled petunias and Calgene Pacific in Australia is hoping for black-stemmed blue roses for the lucrative Japanese market. Researchers at Macquarie University in Australia are working on similar techniques. Revealing the underlying values of control, Quiddington writes: 'The possibilities are endless and may even extend to designer-patterned canaries and cats'.[43]

Internationally, genetic work with animals is proceeding rapidly. It includes the development of transgenic animals, where the genes of one animal are placed into the genes of another, producing a cross-bred animal which may pass on its mixed genetic qualities; and of chimeras in which there is a blend of the genes of two different species in the one animal but this blend is not passed on to offspring.

Research in Australia includes the development of transgenic super-pigs by researchers at Adelaide University under Bob Seamark; research at CSIRO to develop giant sheep by splicing together growth hormone and liver genes; the extension of the super-pig research to sheep so that they would produce an increased wool yield; the extension of this work to cattle to produce more meat on individual animals; and the development by CSIRO through its gene mapping process of a high-meat low-fat chicken.[44]

Australian scientists, like other scientists internationally, are also developing animals for specific medical research purposes. For example, scientists at Melbourne University in association with Genentech of California have produced a rat whose genetic material includes a human gene thought to be involved in heart disease. Rats will be genetically engineered with the human genes in them in order to study heart disease and possibly other diseases such as diabetes. Australian researchers at CSIRO have also produced an animal similar to the British shoat or geep, a chimera produced from sheep and goats; the Australian animal is a cross between a Brahman cow and a Hereford. In this research an embryo is cut in half with microsurgery from both a Brahman and a Hereford and recombined with the half of the other breed's embryo. It is transferred into an animal which produces the chimera. It is developed 'for experimental purposes only'.[45]

In the UK, scientists have not only produced their geep or shoat but have also produced a transgenic sow and her litter.[46] In Edinburgh, the Applied Institute of Physiology and Genetics Research is concerned with developing sheep which will produce milk containing a blood-clotting agent useful to haemophiliacs. The intention is to establish pharmaceutical farms to manufacture animal-produced drugs. As O'Neill reports, 'some of tomorrow's cows could become four-legged factories producing bio-drugs worth thousands of dollars, or may produce customer-designed milk for the food industries'.[47]

Perhaps the most noteworthy development is the general trend towards the creation of animals, particularly rats and mice, which will be programmed genetically to develop particular diseases. These may include mice who are given parts of the human immune system in order that they will 'work like little humans'. They are then models for investigating human diseases. In research involving some of these mice, research groups are injecting mature human blood cells or transplants of human fetal tissue from the liver, thymus and lymph nodes into the mice. The mice bodies are less likely to reject fetal cells. Professor Weissman, Professor of Pathology at Stanford's Medical School, indicates that 'the only limit on the uses of the mouse model for studying a whole range of congenital or acquired defects is the imagination and technical expertise of researchers'. The Fox Chase Cancer Center in Philadelphia is licensing a company to mass-produce the mice for use in research laboratories.[48] Jackson Laboratories in Maine are selling mutant mice at the rate of around 45 000 each week. There are 'tight skinned and trembling mice, hyperactive and lethargic mice, and mice doomed to develop leukaemia and others to get muscular dystrophy... At any moment around 750 000 are on the shelf. And half the strains are available as frozen embryos'.[49]

The first patent on a transgenic animal has now been issued in the US, and patents are pending in Australia. This particular mouse carries in its sex and somatic cells the oncogene which induces cancer. Resulting mice are genetically predisposed to develop cancers, particularly breast cancers.[50] This particular patent was and remains a contentious issue for many members of the US Congress.[51] In Australia there is no controlling legislation and the Australian patent office will grant a patent for transgenic animals if they are seen to represent a unique invention.[52] Since 21 April 1987 when the US patent and trademark office announced that it would grant patents on new forms of animal life, corporations have been getting ready for extensive commercialisation. A patent will allow corporations to own the species for a period of seventeen years. For example, Integrated Genetics in Massachusetts is applying for a patent for rodents that secrete a therapeutic protein in the milk of lactating females. It is considering producing animals that secrete pharmaceuticals in their milk, blood or waste products. The news of the patent possibilities has pleased Don Hudson, president of Transgenic Sciences in Massachusetts, which sells laboratory mice. He says: 'It's especially good in selling [our company] to investors' and they will soon be producing transgenic mice which exhibit features of human diseases other than cancer.[53]

Problems with technology aimed at increasing yields from animals include the possibility that when genes are added to these animals, uncontrollable cell multiplication may take place. This can lead to excessive growth which is detrimental to the animal, causing arthritis or crippling problems in the limbs. It can also cause rapidly growing cancers. The effects on humans of eating any of these products is of course still unknown and only after large-scale experimentation on the consumer public will the corporations know whether their products are safe. To date no government has discussed large-scale studies of populations which consume this food. There is also a danger that diseased animals will escape from laboratory conditions, spreading their disease to other animals or to those in the natural environment. In Australia in 1990, transgenic pigs were sold to the public without the knowledge of the scientists involved.[54]

Of course the gene work being done which injects human tissue into animals has already begun the process of mixing human and animal cells. The fertility of male sperm for many years has been assessed by whether or not they would fertilise hamster eggs. But anxieties continue that science may eventually move a step further by fertilising animal eggs with human sperm and allowing the resulting creature to develop. In 1981 Ford interviewed a number of scientists on this point. Dr Geoffrey Bourne, at one time director of a primate regional centre at Emory University in the US, said: 'I believe it would be very important scientifically to try to produce an ape-human cross, and I hope someone in a position to do it will make the attempt'. He had considered doing the research himself but was concerned about the ethical problems that might arise. Dr John Senner, a geneticist at the Oregon Regional Primate Research Center, was quoted as saying that 'the production of such offspring would be simple' because 'men, chimpanzees, and gorillas have an estimated ninety-seven-and-a-half per cent of their chromosomes in common, a greater percentage than the horse and the donkey, which have been interbred'. Dr Stephen Seager, chief of the Reproductive Physiology Unit at the National Institutes of Health Veterinary Resources Branch, argued that women could serve as 'hosts' for embryos of chimpanzees or gorillas. This would involve flushing an embryo from the apes and implanting it into a woman. When asked by Ford how he would get hold of such human 'hosts', Dr Seager is quoted as replying: 'I think you could find women who are serious conservationists, who want to help animals. After all, there wouldn't be any questions about adoption. It would be pure chimp, or pure gorilla.'[55] The minds of some scientists show no restraint.

Interference with the nature of both plants and animals is justified by the argument that it will increase the production of food which is necessary to feed the world. Yet these goods are produced for sale, not for altruistic distribution to the developing world. It is not the low yield of plants and animals that is the problem, but the inequality of the distribution of global resources. Many farmers are also worried that the patenting of genetically engineered livestock will create a surplus in dairy stocks, putting small owners out of business but giving large commercial enterprises control of these resources.[56]

The assumption behind these developments is that humans should be able to control, use and improve on nature. Bruce Mackler, general counsel for the Association of Biotechnology Companies, argues that man (*sic*) is more benign than nature. He asks, 'Did nature or man create the AIDS virus? Does nature have a Biotechnology Steering Committee? Does nature have a cost-benefit ratio?'[57]

Control at all costs seems to be the slogan. The drive for commercial and/or scientific 'success' blinds researchers and developers to the risks and moral implications of their work. The fact that animals are being deliberately constructed and genetically manipulated so that they will lead lives with disease, pain and disability is glossed over in the rush to control and profit from all animal and human life.

HUMAN GENETIC ENGINEERING

Genetic engineering can take place in the form of *somatic gene therapy*, when new genes are inserted into existing cells with supposedly faulty genes. The changes that result are not passed on to any offspring. *Germ line therapy* involves changing the germ cells (eggs or sperm) or a fertilised egg, which means that the changes to the cells will be replicated in the next generation.[58] Micro-genetic engineering is no longer a novelty. It is supposedly being developed for the purposes of 'curing' and 'preventing' genetic diseases and 'enhancing' an already normally developed person. DNA 'fingerprinting' techniques are already being used in the area of crime detection and immigration, and work is ongoing in the mapping of the human genome, the total human genetic makeup.[59]

Molecular biologists and geneticists are attempting to develop gene probes in order to determine the genetic bases of some diseases. To date discussion has revolved around problems such as sickle-cell anaemia and thalassaemia (both red-blood-cell diseases), Duchenne's muscular dystrophy, cystic fibrosis, Lesch Nyhan disease and manic-depression. Cystic fibrosis, for example, believed to be a single-gene defect, has been 'narrowed to a very short piece of chromosome 7'.[60] This research in the US was carried out with adults. But in England, researchers at St Mary's Hospital Medical School claim detection of cystic fibrosis in very early human embryos.[61] However, the location of this supposedly single-gene defect has so far only been narrowed down to one of possibly six genes.

Similar results were found with fetal diagnosis of thalassaemia by DNA analysis: although one mutant gene has been detected, two other genes have been implicated.[62] *New Scientist* reported in May 1987 that two possible marker genes had been found for Alzheimer's disease, but by November the story had to be retracted because the cause was found to be much more complicated.[63]

The search for the gene for manic-depression is also running up against problems. Named incorrectly in the press as 'the first genetic tag for a psychiatric disorder',[64] a study of an eighty-one-member family in the Amish community in Pennsylvania initially suggested that the gene causing manic-depression was located on chromosome 11, but in fact it was only a marker gene that had been located. Studies on manic-depression in Icelandic and North American families show no linkage to chromosome 11. The condition is probably therefore multi-factorial and may also involve other genes.[65] Scientific reports themselves reveal the inconclusiveness of this information:

> the markers are two genes whose precise location on the X chromosome is known. The gene for manic-depressive disorder is believed to be close enough to these two known genes that they are nearly always inherited together... The faulty gene itself has not yet been identified.[66]

Similar uncertainty occurs with research concerning lung cancer. Molecular biologists hypothesise that there are tumour-suppressing genes which malfunction and this occurs in a two-step process. Vines notes that 'even though researchers have now identified the region of chromosome 3 that carries the tumour-suppressing genes, it will not be easy to find the gene'.[67] Again there may be more than one gene involved.

In 1988 the first medical team applied to the National Institute of Health in the US for permission to carry out gene therapy on adults. This is a study that would insert marker genes into cancer patients in order to trace their route and behaviour. In October 1988 the recombinant DNA advisory committee of the NIH approved the experiment, although an earlier recommendation from the Gene Therapy sub-committee of this committee had suggested that it be put off until the risks were clearer. In 1990 the first trials with gene therapy were approved.[68]

Apart from their claims that they will be able to find genes which will cure diseases, scientists also claim that they will be able to prevent certain health problems from appearing. For example, they are discussing an early-warning system for preventing diabetes. In Australia researchers are looking to find the 'faulty genes' which will indicate whether someone is *likely* to get diabetes. It is suggested that a DNA probe could be used at birth. 'When a child is born you could determine that he has the genes for mature-age onset diabetes even though he might not get it until the age of 70', says Dr Don Chisholm. Though they have only developed two probes and do not know the exact gene involved, the group is pushing ahead with the research, claiming it is preventative health care.[69]

It is disturbing that the research is moving from a discussion of curing genetic diseases to preventing all manner of problems which might arise in children such as asthma or stress. Heart disease and cancer, which have known environmental factors involved in them, are also being considered as genetic problems. Increasingly, health and behavioural problems are being linked to a genetic cause. For example, predisposition to problems in the menopause is now discussed as genetically predetermined. Professor Carl Wood from Australia has indicated that 'emotional and physical problems often put down to stress, or to menopause or to something similar, will also be diagnosed as genetic diseases, and treated effectively with chemicals or gene replacement'.[70] This attitude may lead to invasive medical procedures for problems which may not even be biological, let alone genetic.

Again, commercial interests have become involved. More commercial companies are developing 'kits' for genetic screening—an imprecise science, as indicated above. As screening becomes more and more the norm, it will be handled by technicians and doctors poorly trained in basic genetics (in one university in the US, genetics was covered in three one-hour lectures). Lewis points out that the kind of work needed in order to use the genetic marker system involves the procedure being carried out with entire families. He questions whether practitioners will be able then to interpret the results.[71]

The record of general practitioners' use of other technologies is not encouraging. Obstetricians who used the AFP (alpha-feto-protein) test were evaluated by the Office of Technology Assessment in America and showed unacceptable levels of ability. The OTA found that only 10 per cent knew that if a positive result was found from the test the risk of carrying a fetus with a neural tube defect was less than five per cent. (Ninety-five per cent of the time the cause of the high reading is a miscalculated delivery date, multiple fetuses or some other unknown factor.) Only 22 per cent of obstetricians specifically educated to perform and interpret the test were aware of the high false-positive rate. Because of this ignorance, many fetuses may be aborted on a false positive result.[72]

It is clear that when translating genetics into a testing procedure, scientists are reducing problems to a simple analysis, looking for single-gene causation of possible multiple-gene defects and ignoring environmental or psychosomatic factors.

Once a supposed genetic problem is detected, the question is, what action needs to be taken to restore the person to health? To date, these discussions have concentrated on somatic therapy. David Danks, Director of the Murdoch Institute in Melbourne, argues that it is necessary to evaluate the safety of somatic gene therapy on hundreds of laboratory animals before trying it in humans. He argues that animals so treated should be allowed to live until they die from natural causes because cancer is a primary risk with DNA insertion and the 'development of cancers is age-dependent'.[73] He argues that germ line therapy should never become necessary because the simple procedure of assessing and discarding any fertilised eggs which are not 'normal' would suffice.

Some scientists argue that somatic gene therapy should be replaced by germ line therapy, since its effects are passed on, whereas somatic gene therapy will only deal with the problems for the immediate individual. Germ line therapy, some claim, will deal with cleaning up the human gene pool in general and will therefore be more 'cost-effective'.

Bell has written that 'by the '90s, biotech will be user-friendly';[74] but the Feminist International Network of Resistance to Reproductive and Genetic Engineering at its 1989 international conference in Bangladesh argued that the technologies are not 'error-friendly'; that is, if errors are made there is no way that the technology can be reversed. With somatic gene therapy, there is a possibility of increased multiplication of cells which was not desired and the development of cancer. Once inserted, the genes are uncontrollable and may embed themselves in the wrong place. The inserted gene may be inappropriately expressed, or may affect other genes around it. Retroviruses which are used to carry the DNA in gene splicing may also be dangerous.

Perhaps a more fundamental problem with the work in genetic engineering is that it ties behaviour back to genetics. For many decades now, feminists and many social scientists have been working to encourage a move away from biological determinism, arguing that masculinity and femininity are not biologically determined, that dark-skinned races are not less intelligent than white, and that the poor are not poor because they somehow deserve it. Science has shown the public that heart disease and cancer are related to stress and to diet. What happens to these variables in the great genetic push? Stress should not be dealt with by changing the genetic structure of a human being, but by changing the environment which produces stress and changing the ways that people learn to cope with stress levels.

DANGERS OF GENETIC ENGINEERING

Health risks occur for those who are working within genetics. Although it is claimed that there have been no laboratory accidents for more than a decade in which DNA work has been carried out, molecular biologists at the Pasteur Institute in Paris developed various cancers while working on techniques of genetic engineering. Two of these have died. In a further incident, farm workers in Argentina were infected with a genetically manipulated rabies vaccine which was being tested by the Americans without the permission of the Argentinian government.[75]

The approach of scientists to environmental hazards and pollution is increasingly to determine a method by which those likely to become ill through environmental contamination can be screened out of certain workplaces. What seems to be the ultimate insanity of a science created in capitalism is the argument that we do not need to clean up the environment, but we do need to make people genetically more able to deal with pollution. For example, Professor Werner Goedde in Germany is looking at genetic predispositions in sensitivity to drugs, pesticides and heavy metals, as well as studying those people who may have an increased risk of developing cancer, heart disease and allergies. Paula Bradish quotes Goedde:

> Human geneticists working in ecogenetics and pharmacogenetics, as well as physicians specialised in labor medicine and preventative medicine, should use genetic tests with the aim of achieving maximum protection against damage caused by in-born errors.[76]

But who will control the products of this genetic engineering and its application? Scientists themselves will not have ultimate control. That will lie in the hands of the state and of commercial enterprises, enterprises which are now constructing multinational bases. I have indicated above some of the areas of commerce already involved. The very fact of the patenting of animals and plants indicates that they are being developed with the intention of generating profit, and although the patent office in the US ruled out patenting human embryos, 'its very consideration of the possibility was chilling'.[77]

In 1988, biology boomed in the United States. Government spending on biotechnology increased by 19 per cent to an annual total of $2.7 billion compared to western Europe's $800 million and Japan's $500 million. There were 403 companies involved in biotechnology in the US alone and another 77 companies investing heavily in that field. Sales of the products produced by these US companies were more than $1 billion in 1987. Part of this huge market occurs in the pharmaceutical area, but the up-and-coming field is in genetic probes. Yet research on the use of biotechnology to eliminate hazardous wastes has been neglected, according to the Office of Technology Assessment.[78]

Robert S. First Inc. of White Plains, New York, predicted that the human genetics market will be $48 million by 1990. In an indication of the attitudes of the executives of these companies, Orrie Friedman of Collaborative Research, which is working on a gene probe for cystic fibrosis, said, 'we have 54 markers on chromosome 7. We have mapped it in a way no chromosome has ever been mapped—we really own chromosome 7'.[79]

Many of the companies are intending, once they have found ways of predicting potential health hazards for people, to develop vaccines to ameliorate or prevent these conditions. Ray White, a geneticist at the University of Utah, said,

> There are two levels: first, you test with markers to define predispositions, and having implicated [certain] genes... you study how these genes work. Then new means of invention will suggest themselves, and you market the drugs you can take to mitigate the predisposition.[80]

Those interested in using these predictability tests include various multinational companies and insurance companies. In 1986 it was reported that in the US around 100 of the biggest companies were already using genetic tests of workers' blood and urine to reveal so-called 'susceptibility to harm'. Unions are starting to become anxious that certain employers will screen out employees who are likely to develop health problems.[81]

The applications of this technology may be extremely discriminatory. Medical schools might exclude older students because training is costly if the student is 'likely' to have a heart attack and die young. Airline pilots are another group that could be singled out. Dr Kenneth Pagan from

California has indicated that though this kind of screening is possible, the opposite could also be true. 'In factory jobs for which training was cheap, but pensions were costly, such jobs could be relegated to people likely to die young'. In the 1970s companies began to deny insurance to people who were carrying sickle-cell anaemia and yet were healthy.[82]

There is a possibility with DNA fingerprinting and with the work on mapping of human genome that in future people may be given 'gene credentials' indicating that the person is 'predicted' to develop depression or stress-related disease, or has an inherited disease. Robyn Williams put this suggestion to the Director of the Human Genome Project at Berkeley during a conference of the American Association for the Advancement of Science. The response was,

> yeah, it is a possibility ... they will know an awful lot about people which certainly will have the propensity to invade people's privacy. My feeling about it is that the nett outcome will be much more good than harm, but there is a risk of harm ... You have to make your own choice. I think most people will choose not to go into occupations where they will get a tremendously enhanced risk because of the genetic predisposition. But I think we have to allow people free choice.[83]

Other possibilities include the use of gene maps and predictive genetics during divorce proceedings to ensure that child custody is not given to the spouse predicted to develop disease. Life insurance companies could refuse to allow insurance for those who indicated such predispositions, or could have a cutoff point at which a person was expected to die. All manner of abuse lies open if this technology becomes more widely available. Much of this work will be done under the guise of 'genetic counselling' set up altruistically to assist people to make decisions about whether or not they should bear children—and increasingly which kind of child they *should* bear. The Law Reform Commission of Victoria in Australia sums up:

> The development of genetic counselling and therapy may raise other problems for patients. Pre-natal genetic testing is likely to become more common, perhaps even routine. Media publicity of birth defects and the new technology available for detecting and treating them will increase patients' demands for pre-natal testing. There will be commercial pressure from the biotechnology companies producing testing materials. Physicians may urge that pre-natal tests be undertaken to reduce the chance of negligence suits. New sub-specialities in medicine, such as genetic counselling and clinical and laboratory genetics are developing to serve the new market. Government financing of public health programs may focus on pre-natal genetic health issues. Medical insurance benefits may be conditional upon pre-natal screening.[84]

A number of writers have also expressed concern about the connections between genetic engineering research and military interests. Graham Pearson, Director of Britain's Chemical Defence Establishment at Porton Down, has argued that genetic engineering has blurred distinctions between chemical and biological warfare. The concern is that genetically modified naturally occurring toxins and viruses may be released during warfare. In the US, biological research has been increased substantially in the Department of Defence compared to work done under the National Institute of Health. In 1980 the Department of Defence initiated research programmes using recombinant DNA technology in order to 'provide a better understanding of... [disease-causing organisms] *with* or *without* genetic manipulation'. In Britain there are at least four university departments reported to be involved in Ministry of Defence contracts researching genetic aspects of biological weapons.[85] Who will own the knowledge of genetics?

Some argue that genetic engineering and DNA fingerprinting can do good. McLaren graphically presents the 'pro' case when she writes about the genetic problems of some children,

> [Some] may expect to live for two or three years (as in Tay Sachs disease), for ten or twelve years (Lesch Nyhan) or for twenty years or more but with rapidly increasing disability (as in Duchenne's muscular dystrophy). Some conditions cripple either the body or the brain (Down's syndrome, for instance) but do not kill. Others do not appear until middle age (Huntington's disease), so people with an affected parent may live all their lives in dread of developing the same disease.[86]

An occupational therapist working with children with Duchenne's muscular dystrophy indicates that the possibilities for a fuller life for these children have increased in recent years though she still describes their lives as 'a life of chronic sorrow'.[87]

The prospect of invasive genetic work on people who do have genetic diseases raises the issue of our attitudes to disability in general. Special-needs people are seen either as hopeless beings with no quality of life, or as stoically carrying on against all odds. But these people themselves are pointing out that there are a wide range of strengths, weaknesses and capacities in the so-called 'disabled person'; society often stereotypes the problem.

Alison Davis, born with spina bifida, argues that she is not less of a human being because her legs do not work. She argues that discussing a disability in isolation from the individual who has it encourages people not to understand disability but to abort the problem. Davis argues that one of the reasons that abortion after pre-natal screening is advocated is because it is more 'cost-effective than caring'.[88]

Marsha Saxton, who also has spina bifida, has been an advocate of the rights of disabled people. She argues that the approximately 40 million such people in the US have been silenced. She challenges the following assumptions:

> That having a disabled child is wholly undesirable; that the quality of life for people with disabilities is less than that for others; that we have the means to humanly decide whether some are better off never being born.[89]

She points out that most people have not had contact with special-needs people, because of their institutionalisation, and this distance has created false stereotypes and negative images. Her advice to a woman considering pre-natal screening with the intention of aborting an 'abnormal' fetus is to ask herself whether she has sufficient knowledge about the specific disability itself, whether she personally knows any disabled adults or children, and whether she is aware of the distorted picture which is presented to people of the lives which they can lead. The major issue involved, she argues, is the availability of resources for the parents, the family and the community to assist the child to develop its fullest potential. She writes, 'we will most likely never achieve the means to eliminate disability: our compelling and more profound challenge is to eliminate oppression'.[90]

There are obviously varying degrees of disability brought about by different genetic problems, and these cannot be assessed in any way by pre-natal screening. Discussing the two of her children who were born with cystic fibrosis, Jackie Andrews indicated that many affected children have happy lives and live into adulthood. Her daughter Melanie died at the age of ten after a year of serious illness and mild disability throughout her life. Her second daughter Alex at the age of eleven had just won the medal for her class in judo. Given the opportunity, Jackie would not have opted for abortion of either of her daughters. She says that 'in spite of her short life, Melanie enjoyed her 10 years... and the unborn child, like Alex, may have something to achieve'.[91]

Rather than using technological skills to screen pre-natally, abort and genetically manipulate, we could assist those with disabilities to live a more fulfilled life. The life of the paralysed Christopher Nolan is another example of the achievements possible when loving care and assistance are available. Nolan has produced two widely acclaimed books: his second won the Whitbread Book of the Year Award in 1987 in England.[92] Of course, he needs continuous assistance which his mother primarily supplies; and this is something which should be changed. The care of such people should not fall upon an individual but should be borne by society in general. This would involve the redistribution of resources away from research into genetic engineering and into increased assistance for those with special needs.

In her study of women who have used or refused amnio-centesis, Barbara Katz Rothman cited women who argued for acceptance of the risks in having a child, rather than screening them. One woman in her eighties saw the tragedies of life in this way:

> This amnio, it's just trading one grief for another, it's just a trade, just one for the other. So it would be better not to do it, wouldn't it? You can't take anyone else's pain, not even your children's—don't they know they can't?... One life to a customer, one to a customer. You're alone. Ultimately we're all alone, we're each alone.

Summing up the dilemma Katz Rothman wrote,

> For some people, this is the answer: we accept our children, we comfort them, we do what we can, but we

> cannot take their pain and their lives for them. For others, that is not enough. For some, it is better not to have a child than to have a child that will suffer.[93]

But the hideous irony is that no woman's decision can ensure this anyway. The technology is not failsafe, and cannot in any case guard against disability which is not caused by genetics. In the US, the main predictors of disability and disease in newborn and young children are poverty and the extreme youth of the mother.[94]

EUGENICS

The desire for human perfectibility leads inevitably to selective breeding. As Jacques Testart, a leading specialist in the test-tube baby business in France, says, 'with genetic progress, the way is open for eugenics'.[95] Eugenics was a term coined by Francis Galton, cousin to Charles Darwin, in 1883. The eugenics movement was very strong in England and North America as well as in Germany.[96] For example, in the US in 1910, a Eugenics Record Office was established and had two outcomes: compulsory sterilisation laws and the restriction of immigration. By 1931, thirty states had such laws on their books. Compulsory sterilisation applied to 'so-called sexual perverts, drug fiends, drunkards, epileptics and "other diseased and degenerate persons"'.[97] By 1935 20 000 people in the US had been forcibly sterilised, and the Californian law was not repealed until 1980. Sterilisation laws remain on the books in twenty states.

In Australia, eugenics gained many adherents before the development of the policies of Nazi Germany. It particularly appealed to those who believed that 'poverty and misfortune were the result of immutable weakness of character'. An endowment for mothers was rejected by many on the grounds that it would encourage people who were not desirable parents to breed. 'What the world wants is the sound teaching of Eugenics; healthy parenthood... and not the reckless propagating of a diseased and undesirable race'. Unfortunately some feminists were involved in this philosophy, and Millicent Preston Stanley in her speech to the New South Wales Legislative Assembly in 1927 indicated that legislation should be brought in to segregate 'mentally defective persons, for the purpose of effecting an improvement in the race-stock'. Statements by the Mothers Club of Victoria also followed this line and Mrs Priestley was quoted in the *Argus* on 10 September 1935 as saying at a meeting of mothers' clubs,

> It had been estimated that in one generation mental deficiency would be reduced by half if sterilisation was legalised. In Australia there was power to make the race we wished. It should not only be a white race, but a race of the best whites.

There was a movement supported by Jessie Street, a well-known feminist, to encourage the compulsory exchange of health certificates between people who were going to marry. The Racial Hygiene Association put out a number of posters indicating that preparation for marriage without physical tests at a pre-marital clinic was a sign of blindness. These tests included blood tests, chest x-rays, tests for diabetes and tests for inherited diseases. People were encouraged to take blood tests before marriage and women were reminded 'that motherhood was "not an instinct but a science"'.[98]

In Nazi Germany the philosophy extended from the sterilisation of 'mentally deficient' people to their literal extermination, and then on to the extermination of other so-called 'undesirable' groups, including gypsies and homosexuals as well as large Jewish populations. In his extensive analysis of the Nazi doctors, Lifton points out that 'in the period before World War II Germany had nothing to match the eugenics research institutions in England and the United

States'. What is astonishing about his analysis is the way that doctors involved in this extermination, which Lifton described as 'killing as a therapeutic imperative', managed to reconcile their work with that of their Hippocratic Oath as doctors. One Nazi doctor said:

> Of course I am a doctor and I want to preserve life. And out of respect for human life, I would remove a gangrenous appendix from a diseased body. The Jew is the gangrenous appendix in the body of mankind.

But Lifton is not just talking about doctors through the Nazi period. He writes:

> One need only look at the role of Soviet psychiatrists in diagnosing dissenters as mentally ill and incarcerating them in mental hospitals; of doctors in Chile ... serving as torturers; of Japanese doctors performing medical experiments and vivisection on prisoners during the Second World War; of white South African doctors falsifying medical reports of blacks tortured or killed in prison; of American physicians and psychologists employed by the Central Intelligence Agency in the recent past for unethical medical and psychological experiments involving drugs and mind manipulation ... doctors in general, it would seem, can all too readily take part in the efforts of fanatical, demagogic, or surreptitious groups to control matters of thought and feeling and of living and dying.[99]

Some of the doctors involved in the work in Nazi Germany continued to work after the war and may still be operating within German companies.[100] The experimentation which Japanese doctors carried out on prisoners of war was handed over to the Americans in exchange for an amnesty after the war.[101]

The emergence of genetic engineering has seen similar

attitudes appearing. A former health systems analyst in the office of the former American Surgeon-General suggested that the existence of mentally deficient people prevents the solution of social problems. He said:

> If we allow our genetic problems to get out of hand, we as a society run the risk of over-committing ourselves to the care and maintenance of a large population of mentally deficient persons at the expense of other social problems.[102]

And the retiring president of the American Association for the Advancement of Science, Bentley Glass, said in 1971:

> In a world where each pair must be limited, on the average, to two offspring and no more, the right that must become paramount is...the right of every child to be born with a sound physical and mental constitution based on a sound genotype. No parents will in that future time have a right to burden society with a malformed or a mentally incompetent child.[103]

A survey of consultant obstetricians in England showed that 75 per cent of them insisted that women agree to abort any abnormal fetus they might be carrying before an amniocentesis was carried out.[104] As Hubbard has pointed out, 'in this liberal and individualistic society, there may be no need for eugenic legislation. Physicians and scientists need merely provide the techniques that make individual women, and parents, responsible for implementing the society's prejudices, so to speak, by choice'.[105] 'So to speak' indeed.

Whichever way it is organised, through legislation or 'choice', the outcome of eugenicist attitudes means selecting humans of value and non-value. Who sets the criteria? And what of the role of women, who ultimately will have to carry genetically manipulated embryos to term or who are given the 'choice' of pre-diagnosing the health of their children? Wheale and McNally write:

> The gap between the Daedalean power of this revolutionary new science and technology and our inability to foresee its consequences creates a moral duty which can only be executed when the utopian ideal of perfectability, which is embedded in the scientific endeavour, is superseded by one of greater responsibility and accountability.[106]

To date both science and commerce have failed in being both responsible towards, and accountable to, women.

3. WOMAN AS A DISSOLVING CAPSULE: THE CHALLENGE OF FETAL PERSONHOOD

THE EMERGENCE OF FETAL PERSONHOOD

In an advertisement put out by Hewlett-Packard in *Ob. Gyn. News* in August 1988, a new 'Fetal Trace Transmission System' was advertised. This system allows 'rapid transmission and receipt of fetal heart rate traces—real time or recorded—over standard telephone lines' and is intended to link women in their homes with hospitals and doctors' offices. As the advertisement says, 'hard-copy data can be viewed at different locations simultaneously'. (The woman of course need not be viewed at all.) This advertisement carries a large photograph of a fetus, looking very childlike; the caption in large letters reads, 'Today, Jennifer made her first long-distance telephone call'.[1]

Attributing personhood to a fetus in this way is not an aberration, but reflects the outlook of current medical practice, particularly in obstetrics and paediatrics. The journal *Fetal Therapy* includes in its coverage of research and technical advances, 'controversial moral and ethical issues involved in intra-uterine intervention, the legal rights of the fetus and the new concept of fetal personality'.

Historically men have been fascinated by the developing fetus. In the seventeenth century male sperm was said to contain the homunculus, or the small human being who later became the child; but until the development of ultrasound it was women alone who knew intimately the developing fetus and who felt its movement and its life; men could only experience this vicariously through the shield of a woman's body or through her interpretation.

Ultrasound has now been supplemented by magnetic resonance imaging (MRI), fetal monitoring and fetoscopy. MRI uses a magnetic field to develop its image. Electronic fetal monitoring (EFM) is concerned not with an image but with fetal heartbeat; it can be conducted from outside the woman's body or through direct contact with the fetus by attaching electrodes to its scalp. Fetoscopy allows scientists to obtain fetal tissue or blood for analysis. The fiberscope inserted into the woman and into the amniotic cavity through the cervix also allows visualisation of the fetus and is currently being suggested for use during labour so that every move of the fetus can be measured.[2]

The voyeurism involved in the development of a 'window on the fetus' is explicit in this comment by Michael Harrison:

> The fetus could not be taken seriously as long as he [*sic*] remained a medical recluse in an opaque womb; and it was not until the last half of this century that the prying eye of the ultrasonagram rendered the once opaque womb transparent, stripping the veil of mystery from the dark inner sanctum, and letting the light of scientific observation fall on the shy and secretive fetus.[3]

He goes on:

> The sonographic voyeur, spying on the unwary fetus, finds him or her a surprisingly active little creature, and not at all the passive parasite we had imagined.[4]

The fetus, in fact, is much more amenable to treatment than the woman herself.

> The fetus has come a long way—from biblical 'seed' and mystical 'homunculus' to an individual with medical problems that can be diagnosed and treated, that is, a patient. Although he [*sic*] cannot make an appointment and seldom even complains, this patient will at times need a physician.[5]

Though technologies for visualising and monitoring the fetus are increasingly used as part of the 'routine' of pregnancy and birth, there is reason for concern about their failure rates and their possible dangers for women. I pointed out in Chapter 1 that ultrasound's safety is as yet unproven. When used to screen for fetal malformation, it can be wrong, giving a 'false positive' diagnosis.[6]

EFM is also frequently misused and misinterpreted so that normal births are designated problematic, and unnecessary surgery can result, particularly caesarean section. EFM patterns are difficult to read, it can exaggerate fetal distress and restricts movement since the woman has to lie flat on her back. Moreover, it is used to replace nurses as care-givers, the monitor itself becoming the focus for medical staff rather than the woman in labour.[7]

Randomised trials of the effectiveness of EFM show no impact on perinatal mortality. It has a high false positive rate and 'obstetricians do not always agree about the interpretation of abnormal fetal heart patterns'. Routine monitoring has been shown to increase the woman's fear, which can reduce her blood pressure and slow labour. Anxiety resulting in increased fetal heart rate has been found to rise purely with the entry of more doctors into the mother's room![8] In other words EFM could produce the negative effects which it is supposedly detecting. There is certainly no need for its use as a routine screening procedure. As Rhoden writes:

> The routine use of EFM in low-risk pregnancies is an example of maximum strategy, in that the prevalence of the problem screened for is low, the number of false positives high, and the resulting action often very aggressive (for example, a caesarean).[9]

The risks from fetoscopy are also rarely discussed. As with amniocentesis they include infection, damage to the woman's physical health, and spontaneous abortion.[10]

The importance of these technologies in the development of fetal personhood lies in their making the fetus available for visualisation and manipulation. The results of this treatment of the fetus as both person and patient are complex. It is accompanied by the alienation of women, who now become merely the 'capsule' for the fetus, a container or spaceship to which the fetus is attached by its 'maternal supply line'. This *de*personalisation of women is accompanied by a loss of rights, pre-eminence being gradually accorded to the fetus, almost without exception referred to as 'he'. The supposed rights of the fetus are interpreted and advocated by (primarily male) doctors and lawyers. As Drs Chervenak and McCullough write of the conflicts between doctor and birth mother over fetal diagnosis and therapy,

> The resolution of these sorts of conflicts presents the physician with tragic choices. This is because there is no clearly convincing moral argument that the woman's life is more important than that of the fetus or that one form of serious morbidity and handicap in the mother is more grave than such morbidity and handicap in the fetus.[11]

The mother who is nurturing the coming child in her body and who normally cares for its well-being is not seen to have any choices, tragic or otherwise. Nor is she even cast in the role of advocate for the fetus. Rather, 'he' needs outsider advocacy, establishing assumed conflict between the well-being and rights of the fetus and those of the mother. Elias and Annas recommend that institutional review boards establish such advocates and say that the 'routine use of an advocate for the fetus still seems appropriate'.[12]

Yet members of the medical profession want to have it both ways on fetal personhood. They seek advocates for the fetus when they wish to coerce a woman into a caesarean section, but not when they want to use fetal brain tissue for experimentation. They use terms such as 'pre-embryo' when they push for experimentation and 'baby' when they wish to exclude women from abortions past week 20. Amniocentesis leads to abortion between the twentieth and twenty-fourth weeks, yet some medicos refuse to abort this far into the pregnancy as technological advances allow younger and younger premature babies to be kept alive. They themselves are confused about the dividing line between the pre-embryo, embryo, fetus, baby and child. Definitions depend on the use to which the resulting 'product' is to be put. What they are not confused about is who should decide the outcome in any of these circumstances.

It is no accident of history that the emphasis on the fetus as a patient with 'rights' comes at the time when women are demanding more control over pregnancy and birth, many of them moving outside the Western medical tradition to home birth and to women's health centres. The technologies developed to monitor, save, 'improve' or discard the fetus endanger this control. All the technologies affect the mother, yet the fetus is named as the central character. By giving the fetus rights, medicine ends up by giving it greater rights than a woman.

FETAL PERSONHOOD AND THE LOSS OF WOMEN'S AUTONOMY

That fetal rights threaten and in fact supersede women's autonomy is most clearly shown in the occurrence of coerced caesarean section where women have been legally constrained to have the operation on the grounds that the fetus required it, and in the development of hazardous workplace legislation which tries to exclude women from certain jobs because of possible risk to the potential unborn child. Fetal rights also threaten women's access to abortion—a major issue, especially for feminists.

COERCED CAESAREAN SECTION

In discussions concerning caesarean section the woman is deemed to have prior rights up to twenty-eight weeks, the period during which most abortions are carried out; it is the last trimester which is now a battleground. Many doctors are arguing that it is at this point that the state has a right to intervene to protect the fetus. A number of cases of coerced caesarean have been documented, particularly in the US.[13] In these instances court orders were taken out to compel the women to undergo medical procedures. In two cases women refused to have caesarean sections even though they had placenta praevia (the placenta having grown over the uterus opening), a condition which can be life-threatening for mother and child: one woman in Georgia refused to have the caesarean on religious grounds and another in Colorado was described as 'uncooperative and belligerent'. In both cases the court orders to force the caesarean on the woman were not carried out: in the first case the diagnosis was probably incorrect and the mother delivered naturally; in the second the mother gave in when told of the judge's order.[14]

In another case, in 1981, a woman was forced to undergo a caesarean section by a court order when fetal distress occurred in labour. She was seen by a psychiatrist and was noted as 'capable of understanding the circumstances and making a rational decision', yet the hospital went ahead and requested interference by the court.[15]

In yet another case Barbara Jeffries was diagnosed as having placenta praevia. The hospital obtained a court order making her fetus a ward of the court, legally permitting doctors to carry out any procedure. A month before she was due to deliver Jeffries went into hiding and only presented at a hospital when she was ready to deliver, which she successfully did, vaginally. There are at least twenty-one cases of such legal intervention, 86 per cent of which have been 'successful'. Louise Chunn comments that

> Tellingly, four out of five of those women were Black, Asian or Hispanic, nearly half were unmarried and all were being treated in teaching hospitals or were receiving public assistance. So if you are white and paying your own medical costs, you were capable of making a choice. If you were Black and reliant on welfare, doctors knew best and you better accept that or a court order would soon whip you into shape.[16]

She also instances a case in the US where a Nigerian woman was forced against her will to undergo a caesarean by being shackled to an operating table.

The most offensive case of coercion was that of a woman in the US, Angie, who had bone cancer from the age of thirteen. She thought her cancer was in remission and married and became pregnant. In this case a three-judge panel conferred by telephone and forced her to undergo a caesarean section against her will. Angie consistently expressed her desire to maintain her quality of life until the end and did not want to undergo unnecessary surgery. The fetus was delivered at the twenty-sixth week of pregnancy and died a few hours later. Angie died two days after the surgery. Her mother said:

> We told the judge she didn't want the surgery, that we didn't want her to suffer any more, that we didn't think the baby would live. But they didn't listen. After the surgery and after they told her the baby was dead, I think Angie just gave up.[17]

Constantly in these cases, the law goes hand-in-hand with medicine in privileging the fetus over the woman. Perhaps the most obvious case of the depersonalisation of the woman and the personalisation of the fetus happened in Kentucky in 1984. A charge of murder was brought against a man called Robert Hollis who did not want his wife to have the child she was bearing. He took her to a barn, stuck his hand into her vagina and pushed the fetus upwards with such force that the uterine wall was split and the fetus was forced into the abdominal cavity. A doctor who treated the woman estimated the fetus had been in the twenty-eighth or twenty-ninth week of gestation and would have been able to survive after the birth. Hollis was charged with murder—but *not* with assault on his wife.

> The court further reasoned that since medical science now allowed diagnosis and treatment of the fetus in the womb, the traditional requirement that a homicide victim must be proved to have been born alive was outmoded.[18]

The case went in and out of the various courts but eventually in the Kentucky Supreme Court was rejected on the grounds that the unborn was not a person.

The issue of coercion also arose with the now well-known case of Pamela Rae Stewart in San Diego. She was charged with 'fetal abuse' of her baby boy who had been born with severe brain damage and died a month after birth. Stewart was charged because she had continued to take drugs and narcotics, had not avoided sexual intercourse with her husband and had generally ignored the advice of her doctor. Stewart was initially found guilty of the charge but a higher court later dismissed it.

This case created social debate on the rights of doctors or the state to incarcerate or otherwise control pregnant women. Professor John Myers of the School of Law in Sacramento, for example, indicated that when it is known that a fetus has fetal hydrocephalus which can be (experimentally) treated by major surgery through the woman's abdomen in order to drain fluid from the brain of the fetus, women often resist the surgery. He suggested that the fetus in this case should be treated as an individual separate from its mother.[19]

Bob Masterton, supervisor of the Santa Clara Juvenile Court, drafted proposed legislation which would make the fetus a dependant of the juvenile court 'where the mother's behaviour is judged to be harmful'. His proposal is intended, he says, not only for mothers who are drug abusers, but for those who, for instance, insist on dangerous diet plans or who are 'otherwise physically irresponsible towards their fetuses'. He sees the mother's incarceration in a medically controlled environment against her will as acceptable. Masterton says that 'if a decision is made to carry a child, then the mother and society have a right to ensure that reasonable care is exercised' for 'their' unborn child.[20] Arguing against this, Joanne Jacobs points out that any woman whose child is born prematurely or with a birth defect may be under suspicion. She argues, as do many feminists, that if the state is concerned about the health and welfare of its children, it would fund adequate medical care, food, and the counselling of low-income mothers.[21]

At a panel discussion on ethical dilemmas in obstetrics, Dr Frank Chervenak suggested that the woman who refuses to have a caesarean section in labour when the fetus shows signs of distress 'may not be thinking rationally because of pain and fear of labour'. In this case, he felt, the danger to the fetus should take precedence over the woman's autonomy and he would be prepared to 'restrain' the mother and do a caesarean section. Doctors suggested that a woman could be incarcerated if she smoked during pregnancy or be prevented from physical activity if it might lead to a premature delivery.[22]

In the US, Kolder, Gallagher and Parsons surveyed obstetricians to gather their opinions on this subject of coercion. They discussed the twenty-one court orders which had been obtained in the five years up to 1987. The obstetric diagnosis, using electronic fetal monitoring, in seven of fifteen cases was fetal distress, in three cases it was previous caesarean section and in two cases placenta praevia. Thirty-six per cent of doctors thought that mothers who refused medical advice should be detained in hospitals or other facilities to ensure compliance. Thirty-seven per cent thought that the enforced medical intervention should be *extended* to include other procedures that are potentially life-saving for the fetus, such as intra-uterine transfusion, and twenty-six per cent advocated state surveillance in the third trimester of women who stay outside the hospital system. Only twenty-four per cent consistently upheld a competent woman's right to refuse medical advice. The authors comment that 'the future legality of home birth may depend partly on how issues of fetal versus maternal rights are resolved'.[23]

In her analysis of these events, and of caesarean section in general, Rhoden highlights the significantly higher rates of maternal mortality and morbidity associated with caesareans (the risk of death from caesarean is four times that of vaginal delivery). Patients can also suffer from post-operative infection of the endometrium, urinary tract or surgical wound, and these are five to ten times more common after caesarean than vaginal birth. Other maternal risks include trauma to the nearby organs such as the uterus, bladder and bowel, hernia, bowel obstruction and haemorrhage. Complications may make future childbearing difficult and future vaginal delivery less likely.

At a programme on 'pre-natal abuse' of licit and illicit drugs in the US, Dr Norman Fost discussed using force in medical treatment of a fetus against a mother's wishes. He outlined the 'test for each case of forced intervention': the treatment should only be employed if the fetus was at high risk of serious harm, the treatment posed low risk of serious harm to the mother, there was clear benefit from the treatment, and the fetus was viable.[24]

This discussion appears to have taken place at least a year after the Committee on Ethics of the American College of Obstetricians and Gynecologists had determined against the use of court orders to force treatment on pregnant women against their wishes. Discussions by doctors of this determination indicated that physicians were interpreting the statement according to their own position on coercion or incarceration. Dr Frank Chervenak, for example, faulted the statement for not advocating a more 'aggressive' type of persuasion if the woman refuses the intervention. He suggested enlisting the support of the father or family members in order to be 'helpful' in this situation. In cases of placenta praevia he argued for a court order.[25]

This kind of attitude is also developing in Australia. A South Australian psychiatrist, Dr John Condon from Adelaide's Flinders Medical Centre, has identified what he claims to be fetal abuse, defined as physical abuse, 'chemical assault' through alcohol, nicotine or other drugs, or fetal neglect. He believes that Australia will soon see many of these cases proceeding to court with the babies eventually being handed over to the state. His survey of 112 pregnant women from 'all socio and economic backgrounds' revealed that 18 per cent acknowledged feelings of irritation toward the unborn baby while 8 per cent admitted an urge to punish it. Another 10 per cent had worries of losing control after the baby was born.[26]

These battles over the well-being of the fetus in the third trimester represent a demarcation dispute between woman and physician, with the arbitrator increasingly being the lawyer. One lawyer has indicated that the defence of the fetus might require 'forcible bodily intrusions' into the pregnant woman. Others hold that the woman should be held accountable if she willingly passes on genetic problems or if after prenatal screening the fetus is not aborted if it is seriously deformed. Christine Overall comments that 'what constitutes prenatal abuse is gradually being expanded so that in some cases even a planned birth at home has been described as an instance of prenatal abuse'.[27] Ruth Hubbard also quotes discussions which imply that a pregnant woman is the slave and servant to her child. 'Negligent fetal abuse' is defined in very broad terms. Hubbard quotes Margery Shaw's argument that

> Withholding of necessary prenatal care, improper nutrition, exposure to mutagens and teratogens, or even exposure to the mother's defective intrauterine environment caused by her genotype, as in maternal PKU, could all result in an injured infant that might claim that his right to be born physically and mentally sound had been invaded.[28]

The lists of coercive practices on the part of courts in the US is increasing. In one case in Washington a woman convicted of second-degree theft was ordered to serve the term of her pregnancy in jail because the judge determined that the fetus needed protection against her alleged drug abuse. A judge in Indiana ordered that a mother would have her twenty-year sentence for child abuse reduced if she agreed to a sterilisation. A woman accused of neglecting her children was sentenced to use birth-control measures for the rest of her life.[29] Though there are certainly problems associated with women and their pregnancies in these cases, the precedent of a judge's decision that puts 'ownership' of the fetus into the hands of the court, taking it out of a woman's control, has dangerous implications and ignores society's collective responsibility.

Not all judicial verdicts go against the mother, however. In Canada in 1988, the British Columbia Supreme Court overruled a provincial government decision to seize the fetus of a woman and force her to give birth by caesarean. The court also ruled that the government should relinquish custody of the child, who had been in foster care since he was born. In this instance the woman, whose first four children were born naturally, had refused surgery, but after the custody order was made she had agreed verbally to the surgery while on her way to the operating room.[30]

The debate has considerable implications for women's autonomy. At the moment the discussion centres around forced caesarean section, determined by an assessment of fetal distress or potential harm, but extension to other forms of intervention is possible: fetal surgery is another area where doctors could argue for coercion of the mother in order to assist the fetus. The concept of fetal personhood encapsulated in discussions of coerced caesarean sets the precedent for this extension.

HAZARDOUS WORKPLACE LEGISLATION

The second area where fetal personhood is dominating over women's autonomy is in the area of hazardous workplace legislation. Lawrence Platt said at a Californian Medical Association meeting that a 'detailed job description including such factors as the potential for mental stress and the exposure to toxic chemicals, should be part of the patient history for every woman who wants to continue working during her pregnancy'. Although the findings in several countries linking fetal outcome to work have been inconclusive, it is implied that maternal work is influential. In one investigation in England the stillbirth rate was higher in women who worked, though in a French study the perinatal outcome was improved in children with working mothers. It is argued that women who are physically active and have to remain standing or walking during working hours, for example in nursing, may face an increased risk. Platt argues that 'physical or strenuous work increases the mother's cardiac output, which decreases fetal blood flow, causing reduced fetal growth'. He argues that women who have stress at work may be retarding the growth of their fetus.[31] These suggestions, together with discussions of fetal rights, may lead to women being constrained from working altogether or from working in so-called 'stressful' environments if they are pregnant.

In the US, workers in the auto, steel, chemical and rubber industries have been severely affected. At Willow Island, a plant of the American Cyanamid Company gave all women in eight of the plant's ten departments the 'choice' of losing their jobs or being sterilised. Five agreed to be sterilised. Ironically, the department concerned closed a year later, so the women were both sterile and jobless.[32]

A quote from the US National Council of Radiation Protection, which is a private non-governmental organisation that helps to set radiation exposure levels, sets the tone of 'protective' statement in this field:

> The need to minimise exposure of the embryo and the fetus is paramount. It becomes the controlling factor in the occupational exposure of fertile women... for conceptual purposes the chosen dose [limit of radiation] essentially functions to *treat the unborn child as a member of the public involuntarily brought into controlled areas.*[33]

Fetal protection policies are being disputed in a number of US companies. All fertile women working for Johnson Controls Inc., which exposes workers to lead as it creates batteries, are banned from hazardous areas unless they can prove their sterility. In a court of appeals, judges ruled seven to four to support this policy, but the United Auto Workers Union was fighting this in the Supreme Court.[34] A 'conservative' judge estimated that 20 million jobs were at stake for women because of the hazards of modern workplaces.

There are important implications for women and men in these exclusionary practices. They focus on female employment in heavy industry and ignore other reproductive hazards to women in traditional occupations, for example, in hospital work. They ignore the fact that harmful mutagenetic and teratogenetic agents may be transmitted to the fetus through sperm, they treat *all* fertile women as potentially pregnant and therefore potentially vulnerable, tying women's destiny as childbearers into employment rights. The rights of women for employment and the rights of the fetus become 'diametrically opposed'. So 'the medical profession, along with corporations, has come to assert a "protective" relationship to the fetus, both clinically and legally'.[35] These kinds of practices also do nothing to ensure that hazardous workplaces are cleared up for all workers—including men. (Fetuses can equally suffer damage through their fathers' sperm.)

TECHNOLOGIES FOR SCREENING THE FETUS

As the fetus becomes the primary patient, medicine seeks to exert quality control over it, so technologies for screening the fetus are intended at this stage to determine whether a fetus or embryo should be discarded. The major procedures currently are chorionic villus sampling (CVS) and amniocentesis. At the moment abortion is the widely used ‘treatment’ for any abnormality discovered in the developing fetus. One of the reasons the medical profession has supported a woman’s right to abortion is because there was no point in developing procedures like amniocentesis if abortion is not available.

Amniocentesis involves the withdrawal of cells extracted from the amniotic fluid around the fetus. Initially it was developed to detect Down’s syndrome, but can now supposedly detect around 200 inherited conditions, though most of them are rare. Originally introduced in order to assist women over the age of forty to detect a Down’s syndrome child, amniocentesis is now used for a much broader population of women; the age limit has gradually dropped to the mid-thirties and now in the West women around the age of thirty-three are encouraged to use it.[36] In 1950 there were only a few genetic centres in North America performing amniocentesis but the number is now well over 500.[37] Government estimates in the US suggest that 120 000 are done each year, but the exact figure is unknown because there is no centralised monitoring. This is in line with most experimental medical procedures, which lack long-term studies to assess the well-being of women and their children after use of technology. Barbara Katz Rothman found that women generally use it because it is considered to be routine.

The nature of pregnancy and maternal bonding has changed because of the introduction of ultrasound and amniocentesis. The doctor and midwife used to make contact with the woman’s abdomen and listen and feel for the movement of the fetus; now, the technician or doctor turns away from the mother to focus on the fetus on the screen. The fetus becomes more visible and the woman more invisible. Women talk about bonding with their coming child when they see it on the screen rather than bonding when they experience its movements within their body. They withhold intimacy from the developing child, while they await the result of the amniocentesis which may lead to abortion. Katz Rothman writes:

> A diagnostic technology that pronounces judgements halfway through the pregnancy makes extraordinary demands on women to separate themselves from the fetus within. Rather than moving from complete attachment through the separation that only just begins at birth, this technology demands that we begin with separation and distancing. Only after an acceptable judgement has been declared, only after the fetus is deemed worthy of keeping, is attachment to begin.
>
> Reality has been turned on its head. The pregnancy experience, when viewed with men's eyes, goes from separation to attachment. The moment of initial separation, birth, has been declared the point of 'bonding', of attachment. As the cord is cut, the most graphic separation image, we now talk of bonding... Viewed from men's eyes, the movement of our babies from deep inside our bodies, through our genitals and into our arms was called the 'introduction' or 'presentation' of the baby. Only when we touched our babies with the *outside* of our bodies were we believed to have touched them at all—using men's language, we say of women whose babies died or were given away, that they 'never touched the baby, never held the baby'.[38]

So, she continues, 'the technology assumes and thus demands of women, that our experience parallels men's, that we too start from separation and come to intimacy—and only with caution'.

There are also risks associated with amniocentesis, risks of miscarriage, infection and damage to the fetus;

and the procedure can only take place between the sixteenth and twentieth week of pregnancy, entailing a late abortion which is both unpleasant and more dangerous for the woman concerned. A number of studies report problems with amniocentesis, apart from the fact that it has to entail use of ultrasound. Dr Ann Tabor found in a randomised study of 4606 women, half of whom were an experimental group undergoing amniocentesis and half a control group, that there was a spontaneous abortion rate of 1.7 per cent attributable to the test. Abdominal pain was reported by 8.1 per cent of the mothers undergoing amniocentesis. In a British study and in a study by the US National Institute of Child Health and Human Development it was found that children born to mothers who underwent amniocentesis are more likely to have respiratory complications and to spend a longer period in hospital than those children of mothers who did not undergo the test.[39]

A new technique which may replace amniocentesis is chorionic villus sampling (CVS). This procedure involves passing a needle through the abdomen or through the vagina to collect cell culture from the chorion (early placenta) of the developing fetus. Tissue is taken from the chorion, using a metal tube that is guided by ultrasound. DNA is extracted from this tissue to test for genetic conditions such as Down's syndrome, haemophilia, sickle-cell anaemia and thalassaemia. Its advantage over amniocentesis is that it can be done at around ten weeks and the culture develops more quickly so that abortion can be done at an earlier stage. It too involves ultrasound, to assess the growth and viability of the fetus.

In spite of it being hailed as the new saviour in terms of eliminating birth defects and of being totally safe and accurate, there are problems with the procedure. As with amniocentesis the catheter often has to be inserted into the woman's body more than once and often three times in order to collect the tissue. The technique would supposedly be used by older women and yet advanced maternal age increases the risk of spontaneous abortion after CVS is used.[40] In one study in the Netherlands, older mothers had an abortion rate above 7 per cent after CVS compared with the average rate of 3 per cent.[41] In addition, a number of commentators point out that a chromosomal abnormality detected by CVS at ten weeks might in any case have caused the fetus to abort spontaneously, before amniocentesis was feasible at sixteen weeks.

A comparative study of the two techniques found that the disadvantages of CVS include increased fetal loss and increased diagnostic error rate. Though the authors of the study favour both amniocentesis and CVS they point out that with CVS there is a 2.6 per cent rate of failure in attempts to obtain the tissue sample. Looking at a number of studies they put the spontaneous abortion rate after the procedure at around 4 per cent compared to 0.6 per cent after amniocentesis. Maternal morbidity stands at 1.16 per cent compared to 0.02 per cent in amniocentesis. Problems include the difficulty of obtaining an appropriate sample, the possibility of rupturing the chorion and fetal loss or miscarriage. There is also the risk of infection to the woman. The authors conclude that 'long-term sequelae are yet to be evaluated'.[42]

In another study of over 1000 patients referred to the Genetics and IVF Institute in the US the authors support what they call the safe, accurate and relatively low-risk procedure of CVS. Yet they point out that additional amniocentesis will be necessary in some cases and that the 'exact risk figures for complications of chorionic villus sampling remain to be established'.[43]

In 1986 Dr Aubrey Milunsky, Professor of Paediatrics, Obstetrics and Gynaecology at the Boston University School of Medicine, said he was concerned about the three cases of septic shock in women reported in the United States and in London which had almost resulted in their deaths, because of infection from the catheter; one case had resulted in a hysterectomy. As he said, 'to perform a [chorionic] biopsy and entertain maternal mortality as a possibility lends a completely different complexion to the matter'. He pointed out that 90 to 97 per cent of fetuses with chromosomal defects abort spontaneously and the 'CVS may be interfering with the process by not allowing the body to abort normally and introducing a set of iatrogenic [doctor-induced] complications'. He also documented 'false positive' results—cases of abnormalities diagnosed by CVS where normal fetuses were found after the women had had an abortion. At the same conference, Brambati reported a high fetal loss after CVS of 13 per cent before nine weeks and 17 per cent fetal loss after twelve weeks. As Dr Rodeck, director of the Harris Birthright Research Centre for Fetal Medicine at Kings College in London, said,

> We are on the verge of doing the procedure on thousands of women, most of whom will have a normal pregnancy. I suspect we'll find it safe... [but at this point] chorionic villus sampling is a procedure about which we really don't know the long-term consequences.[44]

These screening technologies make so-called choices more difficult for women. How does a woman choose not to use them? How will a woman be punished if her child is 'defective'? She will be punished by the guilt she will carry, by the recriminations of the medical profession, by the work entailed in rearing a child that is not 'normal' in a world which increasingly gives fewer and fewer resources to those with special needs. These techniques put emphasis on obtaining a perfection in children which is not possible.

As Ruth Hubbard continues to point out, the vast majority of women, left alone, will have healthy normal children. By constantly emphasising the small number of children born with problems as if they were the norm and introducing screening procedures as if all women were at risk, medical science creates a picture of women unable to create healthy children and increases women's anxiety. The economic 'burden' of rearing a child who is not 'perfect' may well be used by the state to justify enforced screening procedures. We can wonder whether the time will come when a normal pregnancy, with no intervention, will be allowed to proceed at all.

TECHNIQUES FOR 'HEALING' THE FETUS

Technology which treats the fetus as a patient rather than discarding it through abortion is also being generated. As if the woman were invisible in the process, doctors are carrying out surgery on the fetus itself. Closed-uterus surgery using ultrasound as a guide is used, for example, to correct blocked urinary tracts in the fetus or to assist a fetus with hydrocephalus (water on the brain) by releasing the fluid into the amniotic sac. Surgeons in Sydney used it to empty a cyst in a twenty-week-old fetus.[45]

The procedure is for the most part unsuccessful. The International Fetal Surgery Registry in 1984 indicated that surgery performed on twenty-five fetuses with hydrocephalus resulted in twenty-one infants surviving; however, only nine of these were felt to be normal one to eighteen months after the birth, three had moderate handicaps and the remaining nine had severe handicaps. Of thirty-five fetuses treated for malformation of the urinary tract, only fourteen survived. Figures in 1987 indicated that about 80 per cent of treated fetuses were surviving but half of them were moderately or severely retarded. In 1989, Hutson reported that of forty-five babies treated ante-natally for hydrocephalus, seven had died and twenty had major neurological impairment. He suggests that the use of ultrasound has 'tempted intervention when it may not have been needed'[46] because in these cases there might well have been a spontaneous abortion.

Dr Kevin Pringle from New Zealand in 1988 reported that his team had saved thirty-seven of forty-four fetuses needing drainage of fluid from the brain but that many had subsequent severe intellectual handicaps. Other children had pre-natal kidney problems corrected, only to have the problems recur three to five years later.[47]

In order to improve their success rates doctors are developing open-uterus procedures, where the woman's body is cut open and the fetus removed (still attached by the placenta), operated on and then replaced in the womb. This surgery is intended to assist in correcting spinal defects and heart abnormalities.[48] In a graphic example of the kind of experimentation on women involved here, Elias and Annas discuss a 1982 case in which Michael Harrison and his colleagues in the US carried out fetal surgery on an eighteen-year-old woman in her first pregnancy. At twenty-one weeks, the lower part of the fetus was lifted through a hysterotomy incision, operated upon and then replaced in the woman's body. At thirty-five weeks the baby was delivered by caesarean section. This operation on woman and fetus was in order to rectify a urinary tract obstruction. Instead,

> the infant had mild facial deformities, limb contractures, a small chest, a slightly protuberant abdomen and bilateral undescended testes. After nine hours at maximum supportive measures, the infant was permitted to die.

As the authors point out, 'the line between therapy and experimentation has never been a completely clear one'.[49]

In 1986, doctors in San Francisco extracted a twenty-three-week-old fetus from the womb to correct a blocked urinary tract. The baby was born nine weeks later by caesarean section to a thirty-one-year-old woman who apparently wanted the operation. The baby had been operated on twice after birth and 'although healthy, he has only partial function of his kidneys and may need a kidney transplant one day'. This operation was also carried out by Michael Harrison, who after considerable experience in fetal surgery on animals moved his work into women.[50]

In one harrowing attempt to release fluid from a hydrocephalic fetus by a brain shunt, the mother described the head as though 'you had taken a balloon, filled it with air, and then deflated it'. In spite of the fetal surgery, the child was born with a facial cleft running from his lip to his right eye and brain malformation which affected all his vital functions. When he was five weeks old he began going into convulsions and died from cardiac arrest. His father said:

> Mark suffered a lot, both before his birth and afterwards. But I felt that if I had asked him, 'Do you want to go through with this?' if he had been able to answer he always would have said yes.

This surgery was again carried out by Michael Harrison: ' "There's no question that ours was a successful operation," said Dr Harrison'.[51]

In some cases a woman is required to undergo two or three placements of the shunt. The babies are often born with additional multiple severe handicaps. Ruth Hubbard writes:

> ... the hazards for the fetus are not just the obvious ones of injury and infection. The problem is that growth and

> differentiation of an embryo is complex and poorly understood. From a biological point of view, it is not surprising that severe developmental defects often are multiple. Indeed, it would be surprising if it were otherwise, since a great many processes occur simultaneously in a developing embryo, particularly in their early stages, and many may also be interrelated. When something goes wrong, the error is likely to find expression in different ways and places and can start ripple effects whose consequences may be manifested in results that appear unrelated.[52]

For the same reason, intervention may inadvertently affect the developing fetus in ways that science cannot understand.

The lack of success of these operations and the dangers involved have led some doctors to call for a halt. Dr Charles Rodeck is quoted as saying that 'the question of whether to treat in-utero isn't controversial anymore. The answer is, don't touch it... What doesn't emerge from these depressing follow up studies is the fact that the technology [in this area] is so severely lacking'.[53]

The dilemmas involved in this surgery are quite clear. Already there is some evidence that the fetus' problem may be as easily corrected *after* birth. There is also concern that intervention allows a fetus to be carried to term which would otherwise spontaneously abort.

The most important point, however, and one which is often lost, is that this work is experimentation on women. Discussions of fetal surgery proceed as if the woman's body is not involved, but, in fact, the interventions are quite drastic. The wall of her abdomen is cut into at a time when it is being stretched by the growing fetus, and it does not always heal well. 'Recovery therefore tends to be difficult and is often incomplete—facts that also affect the fetus'.[54]

The language used in discussion of these experiments gives away the medical profession's attitude to who is the patient and who has the rights in this situation. A discussion in *Ob. Gyn. News* on 'patient selection' focused on how to select which *fetus* to do surgery on. Discussing the practice of fetal shunting, Dr Golbus talked about submitting *pregnancies*—not women—to the risk of therapy.[55]

Discussing the replacement of the fetus into the uterus after it has undergone surgery, Dr Pringle described it as 'being replaced into the best intensive care unit, the uterus', once again defining women merely as mechanisms, as a laboratory. He discussed open-uterus surgery as 'open fetal surgery' to benefit a 'sick baby'. At least he finally managed to name the woman as mother when he said, 'If this surgery becomes routine, then inevitably some mothers will die'.[56]

TECHNIQUES FOR USING THE FETUS

FETAL EGGS

Research on procedures designed to mature women's immature eggs taken from a slice of ovary is already under way (see p.63). Extending his discussions of egg collection, Dr Brinsmead indicates that maturing follicles could be extracted from a female fetus by the fourteenth week, when the fetus contains its full complement of eggs. Miller writes that:

> Thus, terminated fetuses or non-surviving neonates could theoretically become egg donors. The bizarre situation of an unborn foetus becoming a 'mother' could arise. A foetus which was not even born could ultimately have children.

Brinsmead says, 'As long as our work...doesn't require the destruction of human embryos, I don't believe we will see public opposition'.[57]

Research by Roger Gosden in Edinburgh has found that immature egg follicles can attach to what Gail Vines calls a 'defunct' ovary and produce female eggs. When there were *no* ovaries, they developed into an ovary. Gosden speculates that ovaries could be removed from children (presumably girls) with cancer and the follicles stored for use in adulthood. He says that 'the best source for human follicles would be the prenatal ovary'. But the problem is that follicles mainly form in the fetus in mid-pregnancy when fewer abortions are carried out.[58] Is it possible that the scientific desire for eggs might lead to women being encouraged to abort later?

FETAL TISSUE

Fetal tissue has been used from the pancreas (in Australia, in order to assist insulin-dependent diabetics), the adrenal gland (in Mexico and the US, to assist people with Parkinson's disease), the brain (to assist Parkinson's sufferers in Mexico, England, Sweden, China and the US, and Huntington's disease sufferers in Tennessee) and the liver (in France, to assist children born without white blood cells).[59]

Perhaps the most dramatic of these experiments has been the transplanting of fetal brain tissue into the brains of sufferers of Parkinson's disease, a degenerative brain disorder which gradually erodes the sufferer's motor co-ordination, speech and so on, but leaves the understanding clear so that the sufferer is aware of the deterioration. The hope is that fetal tissue (external cells or brain tissue), which develops faster than adult tissue and therefore is less likely to be rejected when implanted in the brain, will begin operating and producing dopamine which Parkinson's sufferers cannot produce.

There are a multitude of questions raised by these techniques. Georgina Ferry summarises them thus:

> A... more difficult question concerns why some doctors are engaging in what is clearly an experimental procedure on the basis of rather limited evidence of its efficacy... three big questions hang over the application of brain grafting techniques in humans: is it safe, does it work and is it morally justified? At the present state of knowledge the answers would seem to be: we don't know, we don't know and it depends on your point of view.[60]

As to whether the technique will work, results so far have been mixed; as an article in *Nature* concludes, the assumption of success from the Parkinsonian experimentation is 'surmise only. Only time will tell what benefits will accrue to the patients. Only when there are large numbers of them will it be possible to judge whether either treatment has general value'.[61] Studies to date indicate that there is initial improvement, followed by a deterioration. Ferry points out that animal studies number only a handful and have shown unspectacular results. By the end of June 1987, the number of human patients with adrenal grafts had already exceeded the number of monkeys experimented upon, 'Yet apart from the Mexican results, there was still no clear evidence that the technique worked'.[62]

The experiment is very risky. Three out of eight patients in Mexico who had adrenal grafts died within two years of the operation. Patients have to undergo doses of immunosuppressant drugs in order to avoid rejection of the graft, and these can have side effects including kidney damage and an increased risk of infection. There is also the risk that chemical imbalance might occur in the brain and there is uncertainty about whether the tissue from fetuses is being placed in the right part of the brain. In some animal studies, grafted material has grown wildly and fatally damaged surrounding brain tissue.[63] In some monkeys treated with grafts the brain also increased its size enormously, so that it became too large for the brain cavity.

One of the main issues for women concerns where the fetal tissue comes from and how it is obtained. The tissue obtained should be 'fresh' and therefore capable of development and function if transplanted.[64] Mid-gestation fetuses or earlier have produced the best results so far in rats, while primate work has produced survival and growth from both viable and non-viable fetal material (a viable fetus being one old enough to survive after being removed from the mother; the non-viable fetus might survive for a short time before death occurs after induced abortion).

Theoretically the tissue can come from four sources: from induced abortions up to twenty weeks, from spontaneous abortion or miscarriage, from premature babies that die or from full-term babies which are dead after birth. In practice there are some difficulties. Early induced abortions are usually carried out by the suction method, which destroys the fetus and confuses the fetal tissues.[65] The fetus needs to be as intact as possible to be of use. Methods which would enable this are hysterotomy or mini-caesarean section or prostaglandin induction which makes the uterus contract and may expel the fetus intact. In Sweden one operation did ensure that the fetus was removed intact and alive. The woman's cervix was dilated far enough to remove the fetus.

These are *not* preferred methods of abortion from a woman's perspective, however.[66] Moreover, it is clear that waiting for spontaneous abortions in order to use tissue is impractical, as it is not possible to arrange operations quickly enough and there is no guarantee that the fetus is of the right age and that its brain tissue will be normal.[67] It is possible therefore that women will be encouraged to undergo abortions which suit the medical practitioner rather than the woman herself in order to maintain fetal tissue intact.

Women might also be encouraged into supplying fetal tissue for specific purposes. They might be financially coerced through the development of fetal farming. If mid-gestation is the best time for transplantation, a woman who would otherwise undergo an abortion during the first trimester might be asked to continue her pregnancy until the second trimester. They may be emotionally coerced by the desire to help a member of their family. Social pressure could be placed on younger family members to supply tissue if scientists' predictions that they can put off the ageing process through the use of fetal tissue come true. (Experiments have shown that very old rats treated with implants from the cells of young rat brains increase their mobility skills.[68])

A number of controversial cases have already occurred. Mothers have proposed becoming pregnant so that their unborn child's bone marrow could be transplanted into another of their children who needs a compatible bone marrow donor. One mother of an eight-year-old child dying of kidney failure suggested that if she became pregnant and aborted, the kidney could be transplanted into the child. A woman with severe diabetes was willing to conceive and abort so that the cells from the fetus' pancreas could be used to assist her own condition; another suggested being inseminated with her father's sperm so that genetically matched fetal cells could be used to treat his Alzheimer's disease.[69] One woman approached surgeons suggesting that one of her daughters would become pregnant so that fetal tissue could be used to help her husband who is suffering from Parkinson's disease; two others (one in the US, one in Australia) deliberately conceived a child to be a bone marrow donor to their daughter and son, respectively, who had leukaemia.[70] What happens in these cases if the fetus is not compatible? Is abortion followed by a second attempt acceptable socially?

Financial coercion of women is also an obvious possibility. Women who are poor, particularly in developing countries, may be open to this abuse. And once fetal farming became a reality, women would be encouraged to relinquish fetuses via methods other than suction in order to make the fetal material useful in experimentation, for uses already outlined or for more trivial commercial purposes. Already fetuses have been allegedly bought by laboratories in order to develop cosmetics.[71] Australian guidelines from the National Health and Medical Research Council developed in 1984 list non-clinical uses of fetal tissue which include the fields of virology, cancer research, biochemical genetics, endocrinology, haematology, molecular biology, developmental biology, cellular biology and immunology.

Because of the concern about fetal tissue experiments, governments are rapidly trying to develop guidelines which will avoid women becoming involved in fetal farming. This is not because of their concern for the women undergoing dangerous late abortions in order to produce useful fetal tissue, but rather because of the developing status of the fetus. Suggested guidelines imply that women will deliberately breed fetuses for sale. British Medical Association guidelines stipulate that the tissue should only come from therapeutic or spontaneous abortions and not those performed specifically to obtain the tissue. The woman must consent to its use for research or transplant and the timing and method of the abortion must not be changed to suit the needs of the transplant. The donor should remain anonymous and there should be no link between donor and recipient. There should also be no financial reward for fetal materials.[72] In the US when news of this research became public the White House drafted an order to ban federally financed researchers from using human fetal tissue gained through elective abortions. This occurred at the time a federal advisory panel was discussing the issue and caused some concern on the part of medical researchers on that committee which had not finished its deliberations. Nevertheless, panel members were also concerned that a woman who was ambivalent about having an abortion might be encouraged to proceed with the abortion when told that tissue from her fetus could be used in important research.[73]

If fetal tissue experimentation continues, there will be increasing demands for more tissue. It has been estimated that a market in fetal cells for diabetes, for example, could turn into a $4000-million-a-year business in the US. Fetal cell experiments are supported by a number of companies, for example, by the Californian Medical Corporation Hana Biologics, on a strictly commercial basis.[74] The medical profession will be faced with a dilemma over the status of the fetus as person or as product for dissection and use. But it is clear that the woman would ultimately be held responsible. That is, the fetus will be defined as useful material when the woman has 'chosen' to have an abortion. Doctors will argue that they are merely using fetal tissue which would otherwise have been discarded.

FETAL ORGAN DONATION

The waters become even murkier in discussions about fetal organ donation. In 1987 doctors at the Loma Linda University Medical Center in the US implanted the heart of an anencephalic baby (one born without a brain, or with only a brain stem) into new-born baby Paul Holc. In 1987 the case of Brenda Winner drew international attention when she decided she wanted to carry an anencephalic baby to term so that it could provide organ spare parts for other sick children. Again this took place at the Loma Linda Hospital which was setting up a system for such procedures. The difficulty is that these children cannot be defined as legally brain-dead. They often have to be sustained on a respirator in order to keep the organs intact and therefore would be legally alive with a still-beating heart when the organs were taken from them.[75] In 1988 the programme was halted after repeated unsuccessful attempts to 'harvest' organs from anencephalics. It was apparently difficult to match the organs with children who needed organ transplants and the organs themselves began to deteriorate, making them useless for transplant purposes. Moreover, since the donor babies were placed on respiratory support which prolonged the brain stem function as well as preserving the organs, a declaration of brain death was ruled out.

The emotional stress on the nursing and medical staff was enormous. Anencephalic children were treated just as any other child would be in the hospital nursery, and it was impossible for many staff to accept that they were only being kept alive so organs could be 'harvested' from them. Inevitably there were inquiries to Loma Linda from some physicians who wanted to know if 'severely impaired infants could qualify as potential organ donors'.[76]

In Australia, transplant doctors at the Royal Children's Hospital in Victoria have been carrying out heart transplants in children. These doctors and their colleagues around Australia are reported as being in favour of legislation providing for the use of organs from anencephalics. Mr Roger Mead, a surgeon, said that 'we have been approached by mothers who have known they were carrying anencephalics, and they have wanted us to use the babies' organs'.[77] Grief, guilt, self-sacrifice—these are powerful emotions which can easily be abused in women.

Michael Harrison suggested that the organs from anencephalic *fetuses* could be used for organ replacement in children with a variety of problems including bone marrow, liver, renal and heart problems. He suggested that fetal organs would not be rejected because they were still developing and that the recipients could be pre-treated with donor cells to increase the chances of the graft taking. He suggested that

> in the future, perhaps the unique immunological relation between mother and fetus can be exploited to facilitate graft acceptance. When the need for transplantation can be predicted before birth...it may be possible to induce specific unresponsiveness in the potential recipient antenatally, for transplantation either before or after birth.

He suggested that labour would be induced and the fetus delivered vaginally. This would allow the organs to be collected without destroying them. He argues that brain absence should be considered in the same light as brain death. He says: 'in my experience families are surprisingly positive about donation; they clutch at any possibility that something good might be salvaged from a seemingly wasted pregnancy'.[78] This was the case with Brenda Winner, and doctors indicate it is true of other women who are carrying such children.

The possibilities for the gross exploitation of women are evident; playing on female altruism encourages women to sacrifice themselves by carrying this fetus to term. Little attention is paid to the pain they must undergo, physically and emotionally. Such proposals underline our inability to accept loss of control and death as inevitable parts of existence.

There is concern about the likelihood of commercial traffic in babies for their organs. In 1987 it was reported that health ministers from more than twenty European countries had agreed to ban companies from selling organs commercially for transplant. This included the organs from both living and dead donors, but it did not include material such as ovaries, embryos and ova.[79] Janice Raymond painstakingly documents information from Latin American countries which indicates a traffic in babies for organ use in the US. Though governments from some countries deny its existence, she shows the links between enforced prostitution, poverty, intercountry 'adoption' and the possible trade in babies for organs. She points out that the exporting of children is the 'primary nontraditional product' of Guatemala, reaping the country more than $20 million profit annually. As Raymond points out:

> There can be no exploitation of children without the prior exploitation of women, from whence these children come... Women are the breeders, children are the product bred. We have here the international harvesting of women and children.[80]

THE THREAT TO ABORTION

The concept of fetal personhood and the techniques and technologies outlined here, as well as abortion for sex determination discussed in Chapter 2, focus attention again on the issue of abortion. Access to safe, legal abortion is essential to a woman's autonomy. Yet there is an important difference between a woman with a pregnancy she is unable to sustain deciding to abort, and a woman being coerced (emotionally, physically or socially) into aborting.

There are reasons for abortion which we could question. Sex determination is one, as Chapter 2 shows. Whether or not to abort an 'abnormal' fetus is perhaps more complex. Should women be part of an essentially eugenic push towards so-called perfection—a state which science cannot guarantee? (Many children will continue to be disabled during and after birth.) Abortion needs to be available to women in this situation, but they might feel more inclined to risk having special-needs children if the community took a strong role in their care. With the increasing interest in fetal surgery and technology, a woman may come under pressure to abort her fetus in a particular way and at a particular time, to provide fetal tissue or organs, or to undergo risky procedures in order to improve the fetus and avoid abortion.

At the moment the majority of abortions take place before the twentieth week. It is often, unfortunately, those who are undergoing amniocentesis who must resort to last-trimester abortions. Benshoof has shown that 51 per cent of all abortions in the US occur before the eighth week of pregnancy and 91 per cent before the thirteenth week; by the twentieth week 99 per cent have occurred. Moving the deadline for abortion back to week 20 as has been proposed therefore would make amniocentesis followed by abortion illegal, since amniocentesis necessitates abortion in weeks 20 to 24.

If, on the other hand, late abortions are allowed, pressure will increase on women not to abort their fetuses but to relinquish them into the care of the state as younger and younger babies are kept alive. As Kleiman wrote:

> Doctors are grappling with whether a child born as a result of an abortion should be given the same extra-ordinary care as one born of miscarriage. Hospital ethics committees are confronting the question of whether late abortions should be moved out of operating rooms and into the obstetrical wings holding the latest life-saving equipment. Women requesting late abortions at some hospitals are being told that a fetus born alive will be given all chances to survive.[81]

It is understandable that with the increased use of ultra-sound during abortion which identifies and visualises the fetus, nursing and medical staff also find it difficult to alienate themselves from the fetus when carrying out late abortions.

Daniel Farber, Professor of Law at the University of Minnesota, wrote that 'abortion is a classic example of market failure'.[82] He pointed out that the fetus has no say in whether or not it will be aborted. 'The adult into whom the fetus would have grown might value his life at a higher amount than the parents value the abortion'. His suggestion is a solution which would not ban abortions but create a market. A representative would be appointed to bid on behalf of the fetus against the parents on the abortion decision; the fetus' assets being borrowed against their future earnings. He suggests that 'if the parents win the bidding war, they could have the abortion but must pay their winning bid to the Fetal Bank. If the fetus' advocate wins, the baby would be delivered, but some share of its future earnings would be paid to the Bank. Funds in the Bank could be used for loans to fetuses, or perhaps even better, could be "invested in embryonic industries"'. Against the argument that the fetuses of the poor would be able to borrow more than their parents he argues that this is not the case because the children of the poor would have potential low earning capacities and therefore the fetuses would only be able to borrow a limited amount of money. He writes: 'Unlike any other approach to the abortion issue, this approach gives full weight to the interests of both the fetus and the parents'.[83]

The technologies I have discussed in this chapter generate increased anxiety for women and increased alienation for a woman from her developing fetus. Now exposed to the various proddings and visualisations available to medical science, a woman attaches herself emotionally to the fetus only when it has been cleared and approved of. Many difficult decisions have to be made, often without access to full information and in a context where women as a social group have less power than men.

Some women have been successfully resisting this invasion. Barbara Katz Rothman talked to women who refused to undergo amniocentesis, Emily Martin has documented women's resistance to electronic fetal monitoring and caesarean section, and there are individuals such as Barbara Jeffries who disobeyed a court order to undergo a caesarean and delivered vaginally. Such instances of women's resistance must be documented. Other women will then feel empowered to exercise more choice. As Raynor Rapp wrote:

> It is important to locate and listen to those who refuse to use a technology in the process of routinization, removing themselves from the conveyor belt of its assumptions and options anywhere along the line. The reasons for refusing amniocentesis are many; religious beliefs, non-scientific constructions of pregnancy and motherhood, distrust of the medical system, fear of miscarriage. The commentary of refusers provides clues to the cultural contradictions involved in the technological transformation of pregnancy.[84]

We need also to turn our focus away from the unhappy and problematic pregnancy, the grossly malformed fetus, the birth with complications; we need to reaffirm that the majority of women carry healthy babies and deliver vaginally; and we need to redefine what we see as good prenatal care. Ruth Hubbard has listed the characteristics of such care. They include access to proper food, housing and employment; understandable information about hazards during pregnancy such as environmental hazards; useful information about pregnancy, birth and infant care; access to healthy and unthreatening places where women can gain non-invasive medical assistance; and access to a comfortable, congenial and safe birthplace. 'Good prenatal care does *not* mean invasive tests and on-going surveillance administered during uninformative and intimidating encounters in physicians' offices or hospitals.' She stresses that we need better services for the handicapped and ill children and that 'the need for such services is immediate and pressing, and they do not involve the biological and social risks of the new prenatal manipulations'.[85]

Medical science defines the fetus as having personhood and claims the right to incarcerate women and carry out caesarean section or fetal surgery in order to save the fetus. Yet when they want to do transplants, medical scientists claim the fetus is merely useful tissue. As these procedures develop, and as science claims it can genetically reprogramme 'problem' embryos, women may find their access to abortion further threatened. They may find that they can *only* abort if fetal tissue is required. If science develops these rights of ownership over the fetus, women's access to personal control through abortion will be fiercely challenged.

4. THE DEPERSONALISATION OF BIRTH MOTHERS: SO-CALLED 'SURROGACY'

> One woman in Texas was working full time, was recovering from a recent divorce which had created considerable debt, and was the type of person who was always willing to lend a helping hand. Surrogate motherhood, advertised in a supermarket tabloid, seemed like the perfect solution. Unfortunately, her heart condition was not discovered by her doctor until her sixth month of pregnancy. In spite of her pleading with a cardiologist to find the cause of her rapid heartbeat and shortness of breath, her appeal for help was never taken seriously. She did not have two hundred and fifty dollars for the heart monitor her doctor told her to wear; the baby broker never offered assistance; and in her eighth month of pregnancy, less than four weeks from the expected birth of the child she had nicknamed Jackie, Denise was found dead in her bed with her unborn son nestled inside her... Her mother Pat is a friend of mine... Pat was the one who received the bodies of her daughter and her grandson to bury on her farm. She never heard a word from the baby broker, or the sperm donor and his wife.[1]

So writes Elizabeth Kane, the first commercial 'surrogate' in the US; a birth mother now active in the National Coalition

Against Surrogacy, a woman who said she felt like a 'flesh-covered test-tube' during the experience. As the fetus becomes personalised, women are presented as less like people, they are dismembered and fragmented. They become eggs, ovaries, wombs, body parts disconnected from the whole person—merely vehicles for breeding babies. (Chapter 6 will elaborate on how language has assisted this process.) The term 'surrogate mother' reinforces this picture. 'Surrogate' means 'substitute' (not a *real* mother), yet the woman is actually the *birth mother* and has a relationship with the child born based on the intimacy of its development inside her body and the relationship she has formed with the fetus and with the imagined child. Men tend to negate this experience, make it invisible and unimportant, because it is so unfamiliar to them.

Some 'surrogacy' arrangements take place with what is called, coyly, 'natural insemination by donor'. In its final report the Waller Committee in Victoria, Australia, said it had been told of a number of cases where women had had sexual intercourse with the fertile husbands of infertile women. The children born from these relationships had been handed to the father when they were born. Both Kirsty Stevens (UK) and 'Jane Smith', an Australian surrogate, produced their children through sexual intercourse.

But 'surrogacy' is more often connected with reproductive and birth technologies. It has moved away from the bedroom and into the laboratory through the use of artificial insemination by donor, or more frequently procedures such as IVF and sex determination. In the USA Patricia Foster underwent sex-determination procedures because the sperm donor wanted to have a son. Mary Beth Whitehead was coerced into undergoing amniocentesis and pre-natal diagnosis though it was unlikely that she would need it. Shannon Boff was involved in a surrogacy case with in vitro fertilisation using a donor egg. The egg was extracted from the infertile woman, fertilised in the laboratory with the husband's sperm and then transferred to Boff's womb. Cases involving the superovulation of women (breeders), using drugs which the reports referred to above suggest may be potentially dangerous, have also occurred.[2]

Nancy Barrass was prescribed Clomid. She was deliberately inseminated with sperm which both the doctor and the biological father knew to be contaminated with a bacterial infection. She was prescribed antibiotics for the infection she developed, as well as Clomid, which resulted in a cyst on her ovary. It seems that she was prescribed Clomid because the infection might make pregnancy difficult to attain. But they did not wait for the infection to be cured, 'he prescribed a triple dose of Clomid and continued to inseminate me'. She suffered unpleasant side effects. 'I experienced dizziness, blurred vision, a severe facial rash and intense pain in my left ovary. I was unable to walk because of the pain'.[3]

This triple mix of IVF, the donor egg and superovulation drugs was also used on South African Pat Anthony, who gave birth to triplets for her daughter, Karen (the children were referred to as her grandchildren). Karen was superovulated to produce the eleven eggs from which the embryos formed and was given hormones to enable her to breastfeed. In the Australian case of one sister bearing a child for another, the infertile sister was superovulated.

CONTRACTING WOMEN TO BREED

So-called surrogacy takes place in various ways: through commercial agencies; through independent arrangements, often contractual with money changing hands; and between friends or family members, often using IVF and an egg donated by the woman intending to raise the child.

Some states in the US, Indiana and Nebraska for example, are dealing with commercial 'surrogacy' by making contracts unenforceable in their courts. In the UK it is now illegal, as it is in the Australian states of Victoria, South Australia, Queensland and Western Australia. Nevertheless, contracts are made. Money may not change hands, but when a woman agrees to carry a child and hand it to another person at birth, she is contracting her body and herself.

The contracting man usually wants control over the type of woman who is to bear the child. This control is enshrined within the contracts. In a shocking expose of these contracts in the US Susan Ince writes that she was expected to refrain from any sexual relations; refrain from smoking and drinking; keep all appointments whether medical, psychological and legal determined by the agency; use only those services provided by the agency; and undergo any medical treatment specified by the 'buyer' or agent. She had to abort if the fetus was abnormal, and if she willingly aborted a normal fetus or refused to relinquish the child the father could sue her for the \$25 000 he paid, plus costs. Both the buyer and the 'breeder' signed a clause saying that 'no matter what happens the company is not responsible'. Emphasis was placed on the woman being 'obedient', and Ince's minimal questioning of the contract was labelled 'selfish' and 'dangerous'. Clauses requiring genetic tests on the fetus allowed for the possibility of abortion if the sex of the child were 'wrong'.[4] Similar controls were placed on Kim Cotton in the UK (before legislation banning commercial surrogacy was enacted in 1985) and on other American 'surrogates'.[5]

In the Mary Beth Whitehead case in the US the contract laid down that Whitehead would not abort unless her health was at risk, but must do so if Stern (the sperm donor) required it, and that she would undergo amniocentesis if he demanded it. She agreed not to smoke, drink alcohol, or use illegal, prescription or non-prescribed medications without the *written* consent of a doctor. Ironically, in order to ensure that Whitehead's husband, Richard, could not be declared the legal father of the child (which was conceived through artificial insemination), he had to sign a clause where he 'expressed his refusal to consent to the insemination of Mary Beth Whitehead'. Thus full and total responsibility falls on the woman. Finally,

> Mary Beth Whitehead, surrogate, and Richard Whitehead, her husband, understand and agree to assume all risks, including the risk of death, which are incidental to conception, pregnancy and childbirth, including but not limited to, post partum complications.[6]

Whitehead took extreme means to avoid having to relinquish her child, but she and Stern ended up in the Superior Court of New Jersey under Judge Harvey Sorkow. Sorkow pilloried Whitehead's character and behaviour as a wife and mother. He accused her of being sly and of using her children to gain publicity. He implied that she would not be able to educate her children adequately because she herself was not educated. He compared her unfavourably to the Sterns, including Mrs Stern who was a paediatrician but who would 'not work full-time because she is aware of the infant's needs that will require her presence'. Sorkow ruled that Whitehead was 'manipulative, impulsive and exploitive' as well as 'untruthful'. He awarded custody to the 'father', in an outrageous statement which placed the birth mother in the same category as a prostitute. In Sorkow's words:

> The fact is, however, that the money to be paid to the surrogate is not being paid for the surrender of the child to the father. And that is just the point—at birth, mother and father have equal rights to the child absent [*sic*] any other agreement. The biological father pays the surrogate

> for her willingness to be impregnated and carry his child to term. At birth, the father does not purchase the child. It is his own biological genetically related child. He cannot purchase what is already his ... this Court therefore will specifically enforce the surrogate parenting agreement to *compel* delivery of the child to the father and to terminate the mother's parental rights.[7]

So the child belongs to the sperm donor but the mother is merely, in Sorkow's words, 'this alternative reproduction vehicle'. On 3 February 1988, however, the New Jersey Supreme Court ruled that commercial surrogate motherhood contracts were illegal, and Mary Beth Whitehead gained parental rights. All aspects of the Sorkow decision were overturned in a 7–0 ruling, except for custody which remained with Stern and his wife.

Despite this partial victory, the outcome was not a happy one for Mary Beth Whitehead. It is also not a happy one for other 'surrogates' who are still fighting their cases in various states. Elizabeth Kane still does not have custody of her child. Patricia Foster does not have custody of her child. Nancy Barrass does not have custody of her child. Barrass did not understand the terms of the contract which were that she would have no legal right to see the child or receive information about him and she was misled by the surrogacy centre about this. She was promised all manner of contact by the wife in the commissioning couple, who assured her that she and her daughter 'would always be part of their family and would be allowed to see our child'. She was promised pictures and letters, yet received nothing after February 1987 when her son was five months old. She writes: 'Now I am not allowed to see or hold my son—much less be any part of an extended family'.

Nancy Barrass relates how she was gradually becoming disillusioned with the surrogacy arrangement throughout her pregnancy and became less and less keen on having contact with the commissioning couple. Two months before the date of delivery of her baby she told them

> ...of my need for them not to be present in the delivery room. I felt no special closeness with these people because of prior conflict with them, and had no desire to share with them something so vulnerable and intimate as giving birth. They responded to my request by saying that their presence at the birth was part of what they paid for.[8]

The control over women in these arrangements even includes reconstructing their personal experience for them. In one 'counselling' session for 'surrogates' carried out by Nina Kellogg, a psychologist working for a surrogacy agency in the US, Becky asks Carol whether she has felt any morning sickness to which Carol replies that she has had a dose of the 'queasies'. The psychologist, smiling, says to Carol: 'You don't have to. There is no morning sickness with a surrogate baby'.[9] The pregnant woman's experience is negated, made invisible, re-written for her.

The cases of independently arranged 'surrogate' agreements do not come to light as readily as those arranged through commercial agencies, but increasing numbers of these cases are emerging. For example, in Australia in 1984, a number of newspapers reported that some women had acted as secret 'surrogate' mothers and given up their babies.[10]

These arrangements often end up in heartache as they did for Alejandra Munoz, a twenty-one-year-old Mexican woman who was taken illegally to the United States to have a baby for a relative. This case is complicated, but amounts to the deception of Munoz by her second cousin Nattie and Nattie's husband Mario Haro. Because they did not have a child by Mario (Nattie had a child by an earlier marriage), the couple persuaded Munoz to carry an embryo which they said would be flushed from her and transferred to Nattie. When Alejandra was one month pregnant they told her that it was impossible to do this and by various means of coercion forced her to carry the child to term. They virtually enslaved her in their household, Nattie parading with pillows under her dress to give the impression that she was pregnant. When the child was born they again deceived Alejandra about the birth certificate stating Nattie Haro as the baby's mother. The situation became uglier when Alejandra tried to retain custody of her child but was threatened with disclosure of her illegal immigrant status to the United States government by Mario. Eventually, with help from other members of her family and various friends, Munoz gained legal assistance and was given permission to stay in the country and have access to her daughter. But the result is that the family is split, and Munoz, who speaks no English and is not well educated, had access to her daughter, but on a limited and insecure basis.[11]

This case also raises the issue of exploitation within families. These arrangements are still a form of contract—women are contracting both their bodies and their resulting children away—yet proponents of surrogacy often term it 'altruistic' or 'family' surrogacy because of the seductive power of family ideology.

But here the bonds are more formidable than money. The currency is love: love and gratitude will be exchanged for the child. Often touted as a truly sisterly act, these contracted arrangements have even more complex problems than commercial transactions. Unfortunately, in our society where the communal rearing and sharing of children is not part of the concept of family, and where infertility is such a painful experience, it is often difficult to distinguish between an act of 'surrogacy' out of love and one out of guilt, even in the closest relationships. In one supposedly amicable arrangement between two sisters entering a 'surrogacy' arrangement, the sister who was acting as the 'surrogate' was doing so because she felt guilty about her fertility and ability to have children easily. The infertile sister had depersonalised her sister to a point where she could say: 'We are just using Jacki as a suitcase really, an incubator to carry it. At the end of the day it's our child'.[12]

In Australia 'family surrogacy' using IVF is being pushed by the medical profession, perhaps because waiting lists for IVF are diminishing. These arrangements could more accurately be described as 'technologically assisted surrogacy'. In the case of the two Kirkman sisters, Professor John Leeton assisted in an IVF pregnancy for Linda Kirkman before legislation making it illegal was proclaimed. An embryo from Linda's sister's egg and donor sperm were implanted into her womb. The ethics committee at the hospital where he worked had refused permission for the arrangement to go ahead. Leeton moved his client to another hospital. There was no ethics committee at the second hospital. In Perth, against the recommendations of two committees (the government-appointed IVF ethics committee and the ethics committee of the King Edward Memorial Hospital) Dr John Yovich went ahead with a technologically assisted 'surrogacy' in which a woman bore triplets for her sister.[13]

There are three flaws in the arguments put by the advocates of technologically assisted 'surrogacy'. These people assume that power dynamics do not operate within families; that a woman is less connected to a child which is not from her own egg; and that genetics determine the most important relationships.

Yet power plays in families are seen every day. A woman can be physically, financially or, most often, emotionally coerced to assist an infertile sister or friend. Once she has agreed to bear a child for her sister, the dynamics of the family make it even more difficult for her to refuse to relinquish the child. What woman would risk losing the love of her family by refusing to give the child up? In the US, Lori Jean had a baby for her sister because she thought her sister would 'love me more and would approve of me'. As she says: 'A sister is the easiest and surest target; the love, identity, intimacy, sympathy and roots with the family guarantee coercion'. In spite of promises, Lori Jean was denied access to the baby by her sister and by a California judge. Likewise, Vicki gave birth for her best friend of ten years; her friend moved house and installed an unlisted number.[14]

The arguments which privilege the egg donor in these cases emphasise genetics as determining parenthood. Technodocs and ethicists argue that if a woman carries a child from an egg which is not her own, then the child is not her own. Professor John Leeton of Melbourne says:

> This IVF surrogacy is superior to any other surrogacy because the child will be totally theirs genetically—her egg, his sperm—and the risk of the surrogate mother bonding to the child after that pregnancy is less... this is the point that everyone is missing, the vital point.

Professor Peter Singer of the Monash Bioethics Centre also hails IVF 'surrogacy' as purer than other forms. Suggesting that State Surrogacy Boards be established, he writes:

> The difference is, of course, that the surrogate who receives an IVF embryo has no genetic relationship to the child she carries. Attachment may still, of course, occur; but it is plausible to suppose that the lasting effects of separation will be less severe when the surrogate has no reason to think of the child as 'her' child, but rather as the child 'looked after' for nine months of its life.[15]

Women's experiences once again contradict the 'experts'. In the US, Anne Johnson, carrying a child created by the egg and sperm from a couple, the Calverts, started fighting for custody of *her* baby before it was born. She lost.

The definitions of mothering and fathering are crucial here (see Chapter 6 for a discussion of the role of language here and Chapter 7 for discussions on mothering). Mothering begins for a woman when she is pregnant and carrying the child through to birth. The fetus that is growing is intimately linked with her body. Her blood, the food she eats, the air she breathes, are all part of the developing child. Male obstetricians often talk about the first time a woman touches her child as being after the birth, yet women know quite well that they have had physical contact with that child for nine months. The important experience that both a birth mother and a social mother (a woman who raises a child) have in common is that they have formed a *relationship* with the child; but the genetic donor has not necessarily done this. Mothering has always been experienced by women in terms of relationship. So we can talk about a man who 'mothers' a child, but we would never talk about a woman who 'fathers' a child.

The reification of the genetic egg donor comes from the old-fashioned definition of fatherhood. Traditionally, fatherhood has been defined as where the sperm originated. If a child was 'illegitimate', it was because no man claimed it came from his sperm. Men can only be either genetic donors or social fathers; they cannot be 'birth fathers'. This is a marked difference between the experiences of motherhood and fatherhood. Emphasising the donation of genetic material as in sperm or eggs devalues the labouring and relationship of motherhood.

The complexities which can ensue from IVF 'surrogacy' have not been considered carefully enough. For example, donor eggs have been used on IVF programmes for many years. If women who donate eggs in 'surrogacy' IVF are to be granted motherhood status, will those women who donated eggs on IVF programmes in the past now become 'mothers' if their egg successfully becomes a baby for another woman?

Who will decide what limits there might be on 'compassionate family surrogacy'? In Rome in 1988 a twenty-year-old woman gave birth to a baby for her forty-eight-year-old mother after the mother's embryo was implanted into her uterus.[16] In South Africa a woman gave birth to triplets for her daughter using her daughter's egg.[17] In Australia, Professor Leeton assisted a fifty-year-old grandmother to become pregnant using IVF though in her childbearing years she was naturally fertile. Post-menopausal and remarried, she and her fifty-seven-year-old husband (also a grandparent) 'wanted a child of their own'.[18] This is the vision of happy families being created by the technodocs.

PAYING WOMEN TO BE SURROGATES

The financial exploitation of women through surrogacy reinforces power differentials between classes of women. Money is not the only motivating factor, but for many it is a crucial element. In one study of 125 women who wanted to be surrogate mothers, Parker found that 40 per cent were unemployed at the time of interview or in need of financial aid. Their family income was not high and they did not generally have a high level of education. Surrogates are often uneducated, seeking a better education for their children.[19]

Few women go through the surrogacy process for nothing. When Noel Keane, a lawyer with a large clientele in the US, advertised for surrogates but could not pay them under Michigan law, 'the numbers of volunteers dropped to almost zero'.[20] Payment of 'surrogates' in the US seems to have remained for some years around $10 000–12 000 for what may be a two-year period of work, including pre-selection screening, a number of attempts at insemination, and the pregnancy and birth. William Handel of the Surrogate Parent Foundation, visiting Australia to investigate the establishment of such companies, said he paid surrogates this amount and paid himself $6000 per surrogate for what he described as 'an extraordinary amount of work on his part'.[21]

In England, an American surrogacy agent, Harriet Blankfield, was hiring Irish, Scottish and English breeders for £6500.[22] Because the babies left the country, the possibility of interference from the mother was reduced. An interesting comparison can be made here with sperm donors' rates of pay at the time. In England men were paid £7 per half hour. If this extended to twenty-four hours a day for a nine-month pregnancy, Kim Cotton, Britain's most notable commercial 'surrogate', should have been paid around £90 000. Like other work women do, childbearing for another is underpaid and undervalued.

John Stehura, President of the Bioethics Foundation Inc., has said that he intends the fee to become smaller as surrogacy becomes more commonplace and as he gains more women from poorer parts of the US to add to his list.[23] Dr Howard Adelman, who was screening women for Surrogate Mothering Ltd, feels that women in financial need are the 'safest' because if the woman is on unemployment and has a child to care for, 'she is not likely to change her mind'.[24] This economic exploitation of women seems not to worry ethicists in Australia like Alan Rassaby who wrote that 'given a choice between poverty and exploitation, many people [women?] may prefer the latter'.[25] Calling these alternatives 'choices' makes a mockery of the term. The attitude condones the increasing pauperisation of women.

In contrast, the contracting men must be well off, as costs to the sperm donor are high. They are usually intelligent professionals in the thirty- to forty-year age group.[26]

In the US the reproductive supermarket is firmly established. These commercial agencies have attempted to establish themselves in parts of Australia and in Germany, where they were rapidly closed down after the Mary Beth Whitehead case gained much international publicity and women's groups demonstrated against it.[27]

The companies running these enterprises are in the business to make money. They are usually unconcerned about the fate of the children born and there is no indication that there is any follow-up of these children to ensure their security. 'Surrogates' are usually under the impression that their children are going to couples and that these couples have been screened by the company for appropriateness as parents. This is not usually the case.[28]

Though few of the programmes screen the contracting couple, many of them do screen the birth mother for her 'appropriateness'. This is generally indicated by her desire to bear children for the 'right reasons'. The women are usually screened to establish whether they can give up the child after birth, but for little else. In a catalogue of 'surrogate' mothers put out by the Bioethics Foundation Inc. in California, women are presented like those in *Playboy* and *Penthouse* magazines. Their photographs are given in appropriate poses, and details of their past pregnancies, income, height, weight and racial origins, as well as comments on their educational levels, expenses and the form of technology they are willing to use, are included.

Nancy Barrass has indicated that there is a lack of legal, emotional and medical counselling to assist women to understand the processes they are undergoing.[29] The 'counselling' which is theoretically offered to, or imposed upon, 'surrogate' mothers is basically designed to ensure that they will relinquish their children, and tries to convince the woman that the child she is carrying is not hers. Handel says, 'They [have] to believe, fundamentally, and completely, that the child they are going to carry is never theirs'.[30] To ensure that a mother is obedient and gives up her child, Handel threatens her. In Australia he indicated that

> if she changed her mind she would be 'kidnapping' the couple's child. He intentionally inflicted emotional distress on the surrogate mother to prevent this happening, by telling her that he would 'destroy her life if she changed her mind', that he would 'follow her for 20 years and that she would never get a house or a car etc. if she kept her baby'... Mr Handel said he believed it was ethical to harass the surrogate mother during pregnancy because the child 'is not her child'.[31]

Elsewhere he has indicated that he would tell a 'surrogate' mother if she decided in mid-pregnancy that she wanted to keep her baby, 'I'm going to sue for intentional infliction of emotional distress, and basically try to destroy your entire life'.[32]

Companies used to think it was better to employ women who were single or divorced, fearing complications from their husbands. But 'now they believe that having a husband may be valuable for support. It may be easier for a surrogate to give up a baby because it is not her husband's'.[33]

Commercial contracts are often in dispute in court, and the outcomes vary. Two cases in 1987 in England muddied the waters. In the first case a surrogate mother and the sperm donor had intercourse until the woman conceived and the woman was paid some money as compensation for loss of earnings. She willingly relinquished the child to the parents who were then allowed to adopt it. In the second case custody was awarded to the surrogate mother. The woman lived alone with a small son and was on social security. She had planned to use the money she earned to bring up her son but two months before the birth she realised she was unable to hand over the twins she was bearing. When she refused to hand them over the babies were made wards of court and remained with her until dispute over custody was resolved. On 12 March 1987 she won custody—but not because of mother-right. The decision was based purely on the welfare of the children. A barrister-at-law, Diana Brahams, commented:

> The award of custody to the surrogate mother in the second case was predictable, though whether it will operate in the children's long-term interests is open to debate. The initial decision to leave the babies with the mother effectively cut out the commissioning couple—or at least saddled them with an overwhelming handicap when seeking custody. The couple might have been able to give the children more social and material advantages, and surely there is something to be said in favour of having two parents? The unhappy father [*sic*] is likely to be the subject of an affiliation order for the financial maintenance of the children he may or may not get to know.[34]

Brahams concluded that surrogacy 'fulfills a need' and perhaps should be legitimated in a non-commercial fashion. Again, exploitation of women and their resistance to surrogacy is ignored in favour of the 'unhappy father'.

Commercial interests will not lie down and take the law, however. David Fletcher reports on what appeared to be an attempt to circumvent the legislation on commercial surrogacy in England. Pregnancies were arranged by an American-run agency which employed the women to keep diaries of their experiences. Lorrien Finley, the American head of Reproductive Freedom International, said that the women were paid for 'taking part in a serious research project and not for selling the babies'. This was a pre-natal learning experiment in which 'educational' tapes were played to the fetus to see if it increased their intellectual abilities. The results were to be donated to university researchers. As Finley said, 'I am paying them to do a job, and it just so happens that if they were not pregnant they could not qualify to do the job'. As luck would have it, there were childless couples in America willing to pay $26 000 each to adopt these children; luck had also arranged that the pregnancies actually resulted from the would-be fathers. The intention was that eight weeks before the babies were due the mothers would be flown out of the country to give birth out of the control of English authorities.[35] International traffic in women for surrogacy had begun.

John Stehura of the Bioethics Foundation Inc. told Gena Corea that he hoped to extend his work in 1984 to women from Korea, Thailand and Malaysia. Since the child would not genetically be the breeder's child, the breeder's race and skin colour would no longer be so important. He intended paying the women only travel and living expenses, saying that they 'benefit from the arrangement because they get to live'.[36]

MOTIVATING WOMEN TO BE ALTRUISTIC: EMOTIONAL EXPLOITATION

Women are often encouraged into surrogacy by men they know. Kim Cotton, Britain's first commercial surrogate mother, insisted she had constant support from her husband. 'He was behind me 100 per cent. Without his support *I would never even have thought about it*' (my emphasis).[37] In the US, Janet McLean, twice divorced and not yet twenty-five in 1981, living with her mother and stepfather, 'was not scrambling for money, but it was an in-between time in her life, and when her stepfather saw William Handel interviewed on television, he told Janet McLean that she should look the fellow up'.[38] The 'support' women receive reinforces the pressure to be a 'good woman'.

The most striking thing about the women who have discussed their surrogacy experience publicly is their kindness and bewilderment at the strength of their pain at relinquishing their children, pain which is not assuaged by their having done something 'wonderful' for another woman.

Surrogates are often said to be 'altruistic'; but this labelling draws on the stereotypical, self-denying definition of women expected within patriarchy. In this prescription, self-sacrifice, in the precise meaning of the word, is lauded. Yet, Mary Daly comments that

> in contrast to male modes of self-sacrifice, which are rewarded with the ecstasy of merging, the self-sacrifice imposed as an ideal upon most women is the radically unrewarding handing over of their identity and energy to individual males—fathers, sons, husbands—and to ghostly institutional masters.[39]

Women are expected to realise themselves by fostering fulfilment in others; to fulfil themselves by proxy. Yet they are disparaged for doing so.

> Thus the female . . . often comes to perceive herself negatively no matter what happens. In a sense she cannot win. If she is too attractive, she may be used as an object. If she is not attractive enough, she may not be desirable at all. If she is intelligent, men may be afraid of her; if she is stupid, she will be treated like an article of furniture. If her sex drive is high, she is a tramp. If it is low, she is not a woman. It is no wonder, therefore, that women in our culture find it extremely difficult to develop their real potentialities without experiencing a great deal of emotional turmoil and stress.[40]

In a world which idealises motherhood while giving it no material or political support, women struggle to gain identity through the role of mothering. Yet in general women are made invisible in the world. Their emotional lives are negated, their work is unrecognised or lowly paid, and their voices in historical and contemporary debates are ignored or have been obliterated from the record. Women are made to experience this invisibility in their core selfhood. To remain confident and positive in the world women have to struggle against anxiety, depression and low self-esteem brought about because they live in a world which has denied them a sense of their own reality. Importantly, a person low in self-esteem is also more pliant, more open to moves which will, no matter how temporarily, raise her sense of self-worth.

The experience of not being real, or not existing, is often expressed by women as they struggle to hold on to a sense of self. Andrea Dworkin points out the ways in which women's suffering and the history of brutality towards women are constantly erased or silenced. Those experiences of women are named as inauthentic by men because both women and men do not 'believe in the existence of women as significant beings':

> And if a woman, an individual woman multiplied by billions, does not believe in her own discrete existence and therefore cannot credit the authenticity of her own suffering, she is erased, canceled out, and the meaning of her life, whatever it is, whatever it might have been, is lost. This loss cannot be calculated or comprehended.[41]

To gain a grip on the reality of their existence women struggle to gain attention and recognition. This is crucial to a sense of identity. In a vignette of what William James sees as the ultimate horror for the individual, he unintentionally writes of feelings which many *women* have had, and the desperation which drives them to accept the socially acceptable identity offered to them in order to exist physically and psychologically.

> No more fiendish punishment could be devised, were such a thing physically possible, than that one should be turned loose in society and remain absolutely unnoticed by all the members thereof. If no-one turned around when we entered, answered when we spoke, or minded what we did, but if every person 'cut us dead' and acted as if we were non-existing things, a kind of rage and impotent despair would ere long well up in us, from which the cruelest bodily torture would be a relief; for these would make us feel that however bad might be our plight, we had not sunk to such a depth as to be unworthy of attention at all.[42]

What we have in surrogacy is a reinforcement of this self-killing in women, of the control myth that women will attain status through motherhood, and a false promise of allowing the woman to create meaning in her life and to gain momentarily the attention of others which is denied her in her daily life.

'Surrogates' often indicate their desire to find a meaning and place in the world for themselves through engaging in childbearing for others. Donna Regan from the US said that 'having a child is the single most wonderful thing I've ever done'. Debora Snyder of Michigan expresses the control myth of motherhood: 'Motherhood to me is the essence of life. Without children, I don't know what I'd have to work for or go on for'. She reinforces the idea of women's endless giving: 'I'd been thinking that I hadn't done anything for anyone except myself and my family'.[43] One surrogate mother who remains anonymous but was involved in a Maryland surrogate parenting company said:

> I have never felt so worthwhile. I have a capability I am able to share, and there is nothing more important than children. As far as I am concerned, there is no controversy. There is no greater gift.[44]

An Australian surrogate who refused to give up her child, known by the pseudonym 'Jane', felt that her motivation contained an element of self-assertion. She said: 'it could have had a lot to do with my own feelings of worth. Maybe that's all I thought I could do at the time'. After a terrible battle over her son which she won, she wrote that 'I now feel that having babies is not the most important thing in the world'.[45]

Women often enter into such arrangements because it is something that they are good at. Bored with a marriage which had 'lost its meaning', Kirsty Stevens in England said that

> her two pregnancies had been uncomplicated, even enjoyable. Kirsty loved the sense of being special and apart that is felt by many mothers-to-be and was proud of the ease with which she had previously conceived and given birth.[46]

In 1987 Patricia Foster from Michigan gave birth to a son in a surrogacy arrangement. She wrote:

> ...you're made to think that you are a saint and that this is the gift of life, the most unselfish thing a human being could give another human being, if you will just agree to do it.

Her fight for custody of her son failed.[47] One woman's statement expresses the continuing need for approval she felt from the director of the surrogacy programme. She said:

> The pregnancy made me feel sick as a dog...I was going through a great deal of emotional problems and admitted myself to a hospital to get some rest. I had to place my children in foster homes for the rest of the pregnancy...I would trust those guys with my life. They

> really care about me, they tell me I'm their star. They're my knights in shining armour...I'll keep trying for them.[48]

Similarly, Elizabeth Kane wrote that 'from the time I was a little girl, I was taught to obey' and that this carried through to her dealings with the medical profession, as it does for many women. Working for a physician and coming from a household that deified men, she felt that 'doctors were superior to everybody...my baby broker, who was both male and a physician, could have asked me to walk over hot coals and I would have willingly obliged'.[49]

Kane was America's first legal 'surrogate' mother, giving birth to a son on 9 November 1980, and was part of a crusade by a commercial company during the next year as an advocate for it. After five years of silence, Kane again spoke out, but this time against surrogacy. She, with other women who were forced to relinquish their children, formed the National Coalition Against Surrogacy in the US.

A powerful example of selfless surrogacy is that of Pat Anthony, the South African grandmother who gave birth to triplets conceived using her daughter's egg and son-in-law's sperm—although she had decided never to have any more children after the difficult birth of her son. At forty-eight she faced considerable risks, particularly after it was discovered that she was carrying triplets, which were eventually delivered through caesarean section. She denied having any maternal feelings for her babies, often described as her grandchildren, saying: 'I don't feel any strong maternal instincts or urges. I am doing this because my daughter, not me, was desperate for children and unhappy because of it'.[50] Ironically, while denying maternal feeling towards the babies, she is the epitome of maternal self-sacrifice with respect to her daughter.

One of the few 'studies' into the motivation of women in this area was conducted by Philip Parker, who works with Noel Keane's surrogate business in the US, screening women who apply to be surrogates, counselling them, and at the same time doing research on them. In one of his studies of 125 mothers he found that many women felt guilty for having previously relinquished a child for adoption (9 per cent of cases) or from having had a voluntary abortion (26 per cent). In a newspaper report on Parker's work, Dava Sobel wrote of a twenty-three-year-old woman who was experiencing extreme remorse over an abortion she had had two years before. She said: 'I killed a baby. Now I could make up for it by giving one to a needy and loving family'. Writing in support of surrogacy, Parker calls it 'therapeutic',[51] and suggests that women could benefit by using surrogacy to deal with feelings of guilt and loss associated with previous abortions or relinquishment of children.[52] (This is in spite of the fact that several 'surrogates' expressed a desire to have their own replacement child to help deal with the feelings of sadness and loss.)

The emotional exploitation of women can also extend to making them feel guilty because of their fertility. As indicated in the discussion of sister-for-sister surrogacy by Timmins, women who experience an easy conception, pregnancy and birth can, and are sometimes made to, feel guilty when faced with the experience of an infertile woman. They may also be moved by compassion. Nancy Barrass has written that her desire to be a 'surrogate' 'evolved out of my compassion for infertile women and my love of children. I wanted to bring the joy of a child to an infertile couple'; Mary Beth Whitehead has written that 'I had always believed we were in this world to help other people'.[53]

The desire for approval is a powerful motivating force. In one case the commissioning couple and the birth mother formed what was described as a positive and strong relationship, although Sarah (the birth mother) displayed an inordinate need for approval, particularly from Lisa, the wife. She wanted 'the attention and the reassurance she gained from those visits and calls. She relied on Lisa to help her through the difficult times when she was feeling ambivalent or uncertain'. In a horrifying statement of self-denial, when she initially miscarried Sarah said she 'was more concerned about them than the trauma her own body was going through'. This overwhelming desire for love and approval exposes the appalling lack of love and attention in women's everyday lives. Sarah even comments that 'I had a much harder time saying goodbye to Lisa than to the baby because I had such an intensely close relationship with her'. She also found it difficult to relinquish the child and 'longs for the baby'.[54]

Janet McLean in North America also miscarried. It took a week to lose the baby and she spent days in bed flooded with pain and feelings of loss; she also felt that she had failed the commissioning couple. '"I thought, Oh my god, what is it going to do to them?" she says; "How are they going to take it?"'.[55]

Though often in commercial setups the woman does not meet the commissioning man or couple, many programmes do encourage this relationship, because the intense relationship formed makes it more difficult for the woman to refuse to relinquish the child. A psychologist for a programme in California says that it will only work if the 'surrogate' and the couple meet: 'it works for us because she cannot imagine hurting this couple whom she knows and likes so much'.[56]

The result of this intense relationship with the couple is often very painful for the birth mother. The couples are either not interested in maintaining the relationship after the birth, or fear that she will try to gain custody of the child. Many of them cut themselves off from the 'surrogate' who had been promised, as in the case of Patricia Foster, constant photographs and letters concerning her child. Kim Cotton tried to send a copy of her book about her experiences to the parents of the child, who were American and had disappeared without trace, because she was 'longing for their approval, deprived of any sense of gratitude for what she did for them'. There is a desire on the part of these women not to feel used and abused, although many of them do. Toynbee wrote of Kim Cotton

> It was belief in that gratitude that kept her going. She needed reassurance that she was not just a grasping, mercenary woman selling her own child, but a generous person doing good to a sad couple. But she never got that reassurance, nor any thanks, publicly or privately.[57]

THE COMMISSIONING PARTY

When surrogacy is presented to the media, the picture is always of the desired child going into the empty arms of childless infertile couples. It does not show the number of single men who are wanting to use surrogacy nor the transsexuals who wish to obtain children this way: in one case a man awaiting a sex-change operation wanted to inseminate a 'surrogate' mother first so that he would be the 'father' of the child as well as its 'mother'.[58] Nor does it show the number of couples who already have one or more children.

It is astonishing how infrequently a childless couple is involved in contracting for a child. Often couples are driven by the man wanting to continue his genetic line. In Australia in 1986 a couple adopting the child of a 'surrogate' already had children but the wife was unable to bear more children. Similarly in their search for the right woman, Geanette and Iain Neill were wanting to have 'a child of their own' despite the fact that Geanette, forty-six, had two children aged twenty-five and twenty-one from a previous marriage. Iain's picture of the ideal woman he wanted to marry was of one who was musically inclined, intelligent, tall and dark-haired—and Geanette fitted the bill. But the picture wasn't quite perfect enough: 'and now it would be lovely to see her hold a child... our child'. He was looking for a 'surrogate' who had no sexual partner so that 'it can be assured that Iain is the actual father'.[59]

The couple wanting the child of Elizabeth Kane already had a three-year-old adopted son; Patricia Foster's sperm donor had three children by a previous marriage; the wife of Alejandra Munoz's sperm donor had a daughter by a previous marriage; and Barry and Adele Cohen had one adopted child while Bill and Betty Meadows had two grown adult children (one killed in a car accident) but wanted two younger children. A woman wanting her sister to carry an IVF child in Australia already had a son.[60] Pat Anthony, the 'grandmother' who gave birth to her own triplet 'grand-children', was doing so for a daughter who already had a son aged three with her husband. The emphasis is on the genetic relationship for *men*. Lisa said:

> I knew how important it was for Alex to have his own baby and I felt guilty that I couldn't provide that for him. I wanted one too, but I had finally begun to accept the reality that I would never give birth to my own baby... and was surprised at how enthusiastic he was.[61]

And as Kane, Whitehead, Foster, Barrass and many other women find, these men will fight hard and long to take possession of 'their' children.

As indicated earlier, 'the natural father's' case is based on this genetic contribution. Yet Tomlinson points out that the 'necessary emotional commitment to the child's welfare' from the biological father is questionable.

> For one thing, he will not usually be intimately present during the pregnancy. He will not be the one lying in bed in the morning, feeling the child kick and move; he will not be the one who takes care during intercourse in the final months; in short, he will not be the one who has experiences and makes decisions that encourage and imply a love for the child that will be born. Secondly, the father's acceptance of the child is conditional on the terms of the contract being fulfilled. Why get himself emotionally entangled with a baby that may not even be his?[62]

Little is heard of the experience of the wife, the shadowy woman. If she is infertile she may have experienced the guilt, grief, anger and sense of loss of control which is associated with the experience of infertility. She may have gone through exhausting years of infertility testing and then treatment. For example in the Australian 'Jane Smith' surrogacy case, Sue Clark (the infertile woman) had undergone numerous testing procedures, an operation to repair her fallopian tubes and two failed attempts at IVF.[63]

Women are often reluctantly persuaded to accept the approach to a 'surrogate'. In England, Kirsty Stevens was a surrogate to Robert and Jean. Robert was Jean's second husband and her first marriage had broken up because of her inability to have children, so the pressure to go through with such an arrangement in her second marriage was powerful.[64] In Australia, Teresa McFadden, who refused to relinquish her child to Peter and Ann, wrote

> Peter felt good about being able to produce a biological child of his own... he was willing to divorce his wife and marry a fertile lady if his wife Ann didn't agree to a surrogate providing him with a child... she was willing... as she didn't want him to leave her.[65]

Wives of the commissioning men may fear the 'surrogate', particularly if they have to contend with 'natural insemination'; the sexual relationship between husband and birth mother. This fear is not ameliorated by stories such as that reported by Lavoie in France where the husband left the wife, having started an affair with the 'surrogate'. Distraught, the wife said: 'Now my whole world has collapsed like a house of cards. Pierre and Lizette are together and soon they will have the baby that was meant for me'.[66]

Women may develop an intense feeling towards the birth mother and work to convince themselves that the child is their own. In describing Sue Clark's relationship with 'Jane Smith', Wiles writes:

> Sue says she finds it difficult watching her [*sic*] surrogate growing with her husband's baby. She admits to feeling envious, but not threatened. 'Obviously I'd like it to be me…It's because I've got those feelings I don't want to be seeing her all the time'.[67]

Yet agencies often encourage relationships in order to make it more difficult for the birth mother to refuse to relinquish, increasing the pain experienced by both women.

The wife of the sperm donor may also be anxious that the child will be taken away from her. She can find herself agonising over the pain experienced by the relinquishing birth mother. Harding wrote of a case in England: 'But most upset was the sterile wife, who being thoroughly maternal herself, knew the agony of loss that girl was going through in not being able to keep her baby'.[68]

The wife is in an invidious position. Her infertility is not alleviated or eliminated. She is left with rearing a child which is often forcibly taken from a woman who does not want to relinquish. She may be left anxious lest the child to whom she gives love and affection might finally be taken from her by the courts and returned to the birth mother.

In a situation of divorce, her position may be tenuous as she cannot claim a biological or genetic connection to the child if the egg has not come from her. In a situation in which she is the egg donor she struggles to convince herself that she is in fact the 'mother', even though she has not carried the child, not laboured nor given birth.

Unhappy cases are already appearing in the courts. In the US, Elvira Jordan reluctantly gave up her child to a couple who had contracted her but whose marriage was in trouble. Six months later the sperm donor Robert Moschetta left his wife, taking the baby. Now he, Jordan and Cynthia Moschetta are fighting for custody. After deciding which woman is the 'mother' the courts will have to decide between that woman and Robert Moschetta.[69]

WOMEN RELINQUISHING THEIR CHILDREN

The creation of children in surrogate arrangements is often likened to adoption. Putting children up for adoption was once part of the control of women's sexuality, keeping it inside heterosexual marriage. Kate Inglis writes:

> Their separation was part of an idealised and fiercely guarded social system involving the expectation that all girls be virtuous, all women be mothers and all mothers be wives. Of course, in reality, they were not.[70]

Increasing community and state support for single mothers since the 1970s has meant fewer white babies for adoption in Western countries, though children with special needs are still on the lists; hence surrogacy has appeared as a so-called solution to the lack of 'adoptable' babies.

Surrogacy differs from adoption in several ways, however. The child is not legally defined as fatherless, 'illegitimate' (legitimacy being dependent on a man acknowledging his sperm helped to create the child). It is often created, not by sex, but by medical means and is therefore more 'respectable'. Unlike the unmarried mother the surrogate is presented as noble, as giving the 'gift of life'; her 'altruism' protects the commercial entrepreneur from charges of being involved in baby-selling.

While being defined as altruistic, the 'surrogate' is described also as 'unnatural' in wanting to give up the child. Therefore, society, commercial enterprises, the state, and the 'father' are all justified in taking the child from her. She is not worthy of the mother–child bond and can be kept from the child. This handy switch in consciousness legitimates the action.

In discussions about potential 'surrogates', agencies and commissioning parties often stress that the woman should be a 'good' surrogate doing it for the 'right' reasons. So, in establishing an agency in Ireland and Britain, Utta Quinton describes the surrogates required as being between the ages of twenty and thirty, in a stable relationship, and having produced at least one normal pregnancy and healthy child. 'They should enjoy pregnancy, have a feeling for what they are doing, and be doing it for the right reasons'.[71] Doing it for the 'right reasons' means not doing it for the money. Although the agencies find it more useful to use poorer women who are more likely to relinquish their children, they do not want money to be seen as the primary motivation. The women also do not want to see themselves in this light, and this conflation of desires leads some women to refuse the full payout when they feel guilty after the birth.

So-called surrogates acting for a sister or friend are doing it for the 'right reasons'. Surrogacy breaks the bond between mother and child, but it replaces it with an equally effective control myth of women's self-sacrifice; endless giving to the point of self-annihilation. 'Surrogate' motherhood is one more assault on the selfhood of women. A friend of Gena Corea says this well:

> The worst thing you can do to someone is mess with the core of her in some way and I think *that* is what is going on in the appeal to surrogate mothers. You violate or exploit a person's sense of herself. I think it's the most horrendous crime against another person. Murder is a crime against the physical self but there is also a long list of crimes committed against the selfhood of women and this is one of them.[72]

There are real problems for women arising from the adoption experience which should warn us of dangers for birth mothers in surrogacy. In a detailed national study of 213 women who had relinquished their first child for adoption, Robin Winkler and Margaret van Keppel found that the effects of this action were negative and long-lasting for many women. Half the women reported a constant or increasing sense of loss for up to thirty years.[73] The grief may be blocked initially but surfaces later, perhaps on the birthday of the child, or the time when a daughter would be menstruating. In Australia, the Association for Relinquishing Mothers (ARMS) has strongly opposed surrogacy.

Commercial companies spend time and effort 'counselling' women to convince them that the children they give birth to are not theirs. The women also expend considerable emotional energy convincing themselves of the same thing. Pat Anthony said, 'I was only the incubator for them to grow in'; Mary Stewart, a Scottish single mother, wrote, 'I was just like a postie delivering the mail', and Australian 'Jane Smith' said, 'I don't think of the baby as mine. The way I see it I'm just a chook sitting on their nest until the eggs are ready to hatch'.[74] Other women recognise the deception and self-deception involved in this objectification: 'I used to call myself a human incubator. I truly believed that what I was doing was more medical than emotional'.[75] As Mary Beth Whitehead wrote:

> I remember the inseminating doctor telling me that I was giving away an egg. I didn't give away an egg. They took a baby away from me, not an egg. That was my daughter. That was Sara they took from me.[76]

It is often during the pregnancy that women come to regret their decision, particularly after the baby has moved. Australian surrogate 'Jane Smith' said that at five months she had a scan and watched the baby move, 'And I suppose that did it. Before, I had somehow convinced myself that this wasn't "my" baby'. Mary Beth Whitehead says, 'It wasn't until the day I delivered her that I finally understood that I wasn't giving Betsy Stern her baby. I was giving her *my* baby'.[77] Patricia Foster wrote of 'praying not to go into labour so you and the baby can't be separated'.[78]

Some mothers, like Kane, Whitehead and Foster, fight their cases through the courts with limited success. Others, in countries where the contracts are unenforceable such as Australia, maintain their claims on the child in spite of enormous social pressure. In 1984 'Willa' in Australia refused to give up the baby after the birth. She said, 'Where there is no real baby, it is easy to be idealistic... I started to grieve when I felt its movements... the only thing a woman can get out of this is money. But no amount of money can compensate for what you have done'.[79]

The couple Willa contracted with felt secure about her relinquishing because she already had six children and her husband did not want another. They commented, 'She said he had said to her he would divorce her if she kept the child. That gave us great confidence that we'd picked the right person to do it'.[80] As Dame Mary Warnock, Chairman (*sic*) of the British government's investigative committee, said of Willa's situation, 'The surrogate mother has got two men to do battle with now—her husband who doesn't want the child and the other man who does'.[81]

'Jane Smith' was pressured by friends and her husband to give up her child. After the first attempt ended in miscarriage at eleven weeks, her husband said, 'these people are so disappointed, we should help them out'. He was convinced that she should give up the child and said that 'he could handle anything but keeping the baby'. When she told her husband that she had decided five days after the birth not to hand over the baby she says 'he was okay, but later, he just seemed to pull away from me'.[82]

Although there are women who claim no problem with relinquishing their children, their stories are punctuated with tears. In England, Kirsty Stevens burst into tears when she was driven to their home by the contracting couple. By the time the taxi arrived to take her home and away from her child, 'Kirsty could barely hold back her tears any longer'. Once she was back home with her husband and her children, 'again she burst into tears'. She and her husband decided to have another baby of their own.[83] Debora Snyder from Michigan did not weep at all until she was in bed alone. 'That night as I lay in bed thinking about her, I broke into tears. I kept crying and crying without knowing why'. When she left the hospital her husband pulled their car up next to the car of the couple taking the child. She says:

> I was fine. Then I looked down at her—I went to get out of the car to give her to her parents and I just collapsed, sobbing uncontrollably. I don't know what did it; I wanted them to have her—I knew I couldn't raise another baby—but something hit me... I wanted to leave first—I didn't want to watch them drive away with her. I had a week off from work and sometimes during the day I would start crying for no reason... I'm not crying any more—I still notice babies though, and I try to imagine how big she's getting—I don't think that will

> ever stop . . . I made her and I made her life—it was worth it—but I wouldn't do it again, because now I know how hard it is.[84]

Elizabeth Kane maintains that 'surrogate motherhood is nothing more than the transference of pain from one woman to another', and Patricia Foster writes, 'Infertile women sometimes say they feel pain every time they see a baby, a child. I'm the one who now looks at every child that goes by, at every crying baby that I hear, to check if it is my child'.[85]

So-called surrogate motherhood is creating our next generation of grieving women.

What of the effect on the *children* of relinquishing mothers? Many of them already have children of their own which is why they are a 'good bet' for contractors. These children are severely affected by the loss of their sisters and brothers. Mary Beth Whitehead recalls,

> I was in the intensive care unit in a hospital in Florida, sick with a kidney infection, when they came to take the baby from my parents' house. The police came and knocked my mother down and ripped the baby from the crib . . . my ten-year-old, Tuesday, saw the police storming our home twice, coming for the baby. She saw this once in New Jersey when they handcuffed me and once in Florida.
>
> It is wrong to hurt my daughter, Tuesday. It was wrong to hurt my son, Ryan. It is wrong that we mothers are not heard because we often lack wealth and education.[86]

A number of women have written about the damage done to their other children through their involvement in surrogacy. Nancy Barrass says that the lives of her nine-year-old daughter and the rest of her family have been irrevocably damaged. Her daughter asked when she returned home from hospital, 'Mommy, if I am a bad girl, are you going to give me away too?' For months her daughter couldn't sleep and frequently asked if she was going to be given away. Her psychologist said that the experience of losing her brother would affect the daughter for the rest of her life.[87]

Elizabeth Kane feels that it has taught her daughters to resist male authority, and to learn what she learned too late: 'My daughters will never play the martyr role my mother, my grandmother and I were taught by our church and our society'. She rages against the surrogacy agency which did not warn her of the effect that surrogacy would have on her children. The legacy for Kane is a rift with one of her daughters and her son, four and a half at the time, has needed therapy because of nightmares caused by grief and loss. He has fears of catastrophe separating him from his mother and at thirteen is 'still a clinging, fearful child'. The epilogue to Kane's book *Birth Mother* catalogues the deeply disturbing effects of the loss of her son through surrogacy on her other children.[88]

Australian surrogate 'Jane Smith' went through a different but equally painful experience. Her relationship with one of her daughters, a teenager, suffered because of her decision to *keep* her son: 'she locked herself in the bathroom and threatened to leave home. I suppose she has turned fairly rebellious as a result of that. It was a terrible age for such a thing to happen'.[89]

Perhaps one of the most moving accounts comes from Patricia Foster, who feels that her family was ruined by the whole experience. She is particularly concerned about her eleven-year-old daughter who kept having nightmares after her brother Andrew was born and taken from her. Her daughter wrote the story finally as a composition for school calling it 'Mrs Bates and the Group', Bates being the pseudonym used for the wife of the sperm donor. The nightmare goes as follows:

> One day Holly, my brother Andrew and me, we were all at the park. Then there was four cars that went by slow. The first car looked like Mrs. Bates's car so we got up and went to a different side. They went to the side we were at. Then we went to another side. They went there too. So Holly, my brother and I went down South Grove and we were at the end of the street. There were people coming down both ways. They had masks on so we couldn't see who it was so we had to go on Willow Beach... They tried to get Andrew. They wanted to get Andrew and keep him. They got him from me. They got off the beach and so did we. We never got to see him again. It was Mrs. Bates and the Group.[90]

Surrogacy may be creating a whole generation of grieving children.

THE CHILDREN BORN

No discussion of surrogacy can ignore the fact that children have been created who will one day be adults with their own views about how they were created. We cannot estimate what the impact on them will be of feeling that they were a commodity; that money was exchanged for them at birth; and in many cases that their birth mothers were *forced* to give them up. Moreover, we can envisage pressure on these children to satisfy the parent: 'It is human nature that when one pays money, one expects value'.[91]

Problems will develop when a child is born 'imperfect'. A number of cases have arisen in America where a child was born deformed or disabled and the contracting sperm donor refused to accept it. The most notable of these was the Stiver case where a very public disagreement went on about the fate of a child born with microcephaly, indicating severe retardation and possibly a short life. In the course of investigations it was found that the 'surrogate' had had sexual relations with her husband and the child was probably that of her husband rather than the sperm donor. After both parties initially rejected the child the 'surrogate' and her husband were obliged to take him.[92] But 'imperfect' could mean the wrong sex. A case occurred in Taiwan in 1985 in which a man hired a surrogate to produce a boy. When she produced a girl he attempted to sue her.[93]

And finally, many of those born through a surrogacy arrangement will be deprived of knowledge about their brothers and sisters for whom they may later begin a search. The experience of adoption has indicated that many people want to know their genetic origins, and find out why their mothers relinquished them and thereby to overcome a sense of rejection.

In discussing the experience of adults who are born through donor sperm insemination, Emma May Valardi, who founded the international Soundex Reunion Registry in 1974, a non-profit group aiming to match children and biological parents they have never met, has spoken of the resentment some of these adults feel: 'Many of the children of artificial insemination feel used... they feel that half of their heritage is missing. They feel they have a right to recorded genetic information'.[94]

In recent years society has moved to stop lying to children about their origins, changing adoption laws to make information available to adults who were adopted as children, and in some countries enforcing honesty in AID programmes.[95] Evidence coming from adult AID children is mixed. Clamar cites an adult who knew of her AID origins from childhood on and writes that:

> Knowing about my AID origin did nothing to alter my feelings for my family. Instead I felt grateful for the trouble they had taken to give me life. And they had given me such a strong set of roots, a rich and colourful

> heritage, a sense of being loved. With their adventure in biology, my parents had opened up the fairly rigid culture they had brought with them to this country. The secret knowledge of my 'differentness' and my sister's may have helped our parents accept . . . the few deviations from their norms that we argued for.[96]

Compare this with the anger and frustration of other adults like Suzanne Rubin:

> Artificial insemination sounds wonderful in the text-books, but what it can do to human lives is something else. By encouraging very young, very immature and very shortsighted males to become sperm donors, you are creating countless triads of husband and wife and donor. Unfortunately the missing component is the child. No-one considers how the child feels when she finds that her natural father was a $25 cup of sperm. The fantasies revolve around what the donor was thinking of when he was filling the cup. There is no passion, no human contact in such a union; such cold calculation and manipulation of another person's life. And for those of you who feel that a healthy family relationship can be built around a foundation of deliberate lies, I would wonder what fantasy land you have been living in.[97]

But donor insemination seems simplistic compared to the variations in genetic donation now being carried out. Will children feel differently if the woman who gave birth to them was not their genetic donor? Will they feel a lack of continuity in the sense of being genetically related to the mother who rears them but biologically related to their birth mother? Whatever the outcome, there will be many children who will experience a profound sense of confusion about their origins. There will be many who will resent the abuse of their mothers as surrogates.

What will happen if these families end up in divorce? Will the sperm donor once again have prior rights over 'his' children at the expense of the social mother? Will her lack of biological and genetic connection render the woman again powerless in front of the courts? The tragedy of these cases of dispute await us. But it is certainly true that the children 'must be considered part of a massive social experiment for which they have not volunteered'.[98]

THE FUTURE: DEAD 'MOTHERS'?

If women have been classed now merely as 'reproductive vehicles', birth mothers with no identity apart from being 'a suitcase really' in which to carry the child, how far can they be pushed into invisibility? How far will scientists go in order to prove that a living woman is not a necessary element in the creation of human life?

'Surrogate' mothers cause trouble, make demands, refuse to give up their children, and drag sperm donors and commercial agencies into long and costly legal battles. Periodically discussions come to notice of the possibility of using neomorts (the newly dead) as 'surrogates'. What are the precedents for this?

There are over a dozen documented cases of women defined as brain-dead being kept alive for the sake of the fetus they were carrying. In one such case in Georgia, Donna Piazzi, twenty-five-years-old and twenty weeks pregnant, was admitted to hospital having been found in a rest room unconscious. She was pronounced brain-dead, possibly from a drug overdose. Her husband, Robert Piazzi, wanted her life-support system turned off after she was declared brain-dead. Her boyfriend, David Hadden, claimed that he was the 'father' of the fetus. He demanded that the woman be kept on life-support systems until the fetus was viable; that is, able to survive outside the woman's body.

Judge William Fleming of the Superior Court granted the hospital's request that the woman be maintained on life-support, an incubator for this fetus. The woman was kept on life-support systems for five weeks while the legal wrangle went on. The baby was delivered by caesarean section but died thirty-two hours later, the same drug overdose that killed his mother resulted in multiple organ failure. He was also fifteen weeks premature and most of his organs were not fully developed.

A notable aspect of this case was the debate which took place between the two men, husband and lover, over the ownership of the fetus. Although Robert Piazzi had not at first argued the case that he was the father of the fetus, it seems he may have been preparing to argue for custody. The legal discussion was also interesting. Involved were an attorney for the hospital, one representing the fetus, one representing the Department of Human Resources as the protector of children in the State, and we can only suppose one for the husband and one for the lover. The hospital's petition included the statement that 'although not probable, there exists a medical possibility that Donna Piazzi's body can remain functioning until the point that the fetus would be viable'. The court-appointed lawyer representing the fetus said, 'If the baby dies, you're no worse off than had they gone ahead and terminated the life-support system'.[99] The attorney for the hospital said, 'Tragically, Mrs. Piazzi is dead. She has no more right of privacy, so it stands that the State may intervene'. In an ironic twist, hospital officials released their statement but refused to comment further because they said details of how or when Mrs Piazzi might 'give birth would violate a patient's right to privacy'. So who is the patient here? Can a person have no right to privacy, yet a right to privacy? Or is the fetus the patient? These contradictions have not been addressed. Nor has the obvious use of a dead woman for the purposes of satisfying male genetic continuity.[100]

In a second case in California, Marie Odette Henderson went into a coma in hospital after surgery for a brain tumour. Aged thirty-four, she was twenty-six weeks pregnant. Her parents asked doctors to disconnect her from her respirator. But her lover, Derek Poole, contested this and the court named him as a guardian of the fetus. In an out-of-court settlement Henderson's parents allowed him to remain the guardian of the child after it was born. Marie's body was kept alive with heart-lung support for seven and a half weeks. The baby was 'born' two months prematurely but survived and after one year appeared in 1987 to be healthy and normal. As part of the procedure of keeping Michele Poole alive, nurses played music and moved the fetus constantly to trick it into thinking that the mother was still alive. Poole did not intend to rear the child himself and the decision was that 'she will live with Poole's sister, who has three daughters of her own'.[101]

In a third case, Deborah Bell in London, aged twenty-four, was admitted to hospital after a severe brain haemorrhage. She was kept on a life-support system for five weeks after being declared clinically brain-dead and in a coma. Doctors did not carry out the tests required to establish whether Deborah was brain-dead 'so as not to endanger her unborn baby'. The baby was taken by caesarean section in the twenty-eighth week and was said to have a good chance of survival. After the baby was taken from her, her life-support system was turned off and she died.[102]

These women we assume were pregnant through normal means and in due course would have carried their children to term. What these cases indicate is the desperation of men to ensure they possess their potential children; the ability of men to take these cases to court claiming ownership of the woman's body as vessel and therefore the fetus within it despite the wishes of, for example, the parents of a woman; and the refusal to accept mortality.

No consideration is given to the experience of a child in being born from a dead mother. There is no way to assess the psychological impact on a child who was tricked into thinking that its mother was alive and walking around for a couple of months before 'birth' (caesarean delivery from a dead woman can hardly be called birth).

But what are the implications here for 'surrogacy'? More and more debate is taking place about the use of neomorts or brain-dead humans. Women's reproductive capacity is one of the issues at stake. As the Piazzi case indicated, some doctors are beginning to allow people the right to human dignity only if they are brain-alive. It is not beyond medical science to suggest using brain-dead women as surrogates. They could also be used as egg donors. In discussing the use of neomorts with Professor David Smith from Nashville, Calvin Miller raised this issue among others. He then looked at the Australian situation and considered whether or not a neomort could legally be used for surrogacy. He writes:

> Could a female neomort be used for a surrogate pregnancy? Legally, perhaps yes. In the Victorian Infertility (Medical Procedures) Act 1984, which forbids human surrogacy, the words 'mother, person, woman' are used, but a neomort would be none of those —she would be a corpse, a pregnancy machine. Some argue that a surrogate neomort would be an acceptable alternative because the neomort 'mother' could not try to claim her offspring. And could a female neomort be used as an egg donor, thus having children despite death?

In response to these suggestions David Smith hesitates then says 'Hmmm, yes, well... all types of scenarios could be proposed. These issues would have to be tackled by Ethics Review Boards within institutions'.[103]

In Australia, a bioethicist, Dr Paul Gerber from the University of Queensland, reportedly described the use of neomort women as 'surrogates' as 'innovative and ethical'. A specialist in reproductive physiology at Monash University is reported as saying that 'I can't see any reason why the pregnancy shouldn't go ahead normally, as long as the *female incubator* is receiving the appropriate nutrients and care' (my emphasis). Dr Gerber reportedly said, 'It's a wonderful solution for the problems posed by surrogacy, and a magnificent use of a corpse. It has my complete support'.[104]

PART 2

Setting The Context For Reproductive Control

In the time that passes between the writing of this book and its publication, technology will have continued to move us further and further away from the ideas and understandings of reproduction which were the basis of society before the intervention of reproductive and genetic engineering. We need a framework into which to place these changes, a framework based on an understanding of how power works and who gains from this technology, a framework to help us to form sound judgements about its usefulness and morality.

This section of the book looks first at the values of medical science and its relationship to women and to commerce within patriarchal societies. Why would medical researchers continue to administer drugs to women which can be so dangerous? Why would they want to encourage women to believe that birth mothers are not mothers at all?

I will consider the way scientists, and often the media, have used language to influence representations of women and to depersonalise them. I will analyse the ideology of motherhood, and how it exacerbates the pain of infertility.

Proponents of reproductive and genetic engineering often argue that individuals in our society are free to choose these technologies and procedures or to reject them. They argue that women already do choose to use them. This raises the issue of 'choice' itself and a questioning of the values upon which our society is built: can people make 'free choice'?

These issues are crucial to the current debates. With the understanding gleaned from these analyses, we are equipped to understand new technologies as they emerge, to evaluate them in a social and political context and, I hope, to argue forcibly against the proponents of unqualified technological control.

5. THE VALUES OF MEDICAL SCIENCE

THE MASCULINE VALUES UNDERLYING SCIENCE

Science has been viewed as epitomising 'manly' characteristics: reason and objectivity. It has been 'defined as *the* expression of the male mind: dispassionate, objective, impersonal, transcendent. The female mind—'untamed, emotional, subjective, personal', says Ruth Bleier, 'is incompatible with science'.[1] In fact, history has shown post-sixteenth-century science to be primarily irrational, at times sadistic and often used to suppress those with less power.[2] Yet this way of knowing is construed as superior to other ways of knowing, and the daily experiences of women (and men) are thereby devalued and invalidated.[3] In reproductive technology, for example, women's experiences and responses about the side effects of drugs are ignored.

Bias intrudes into science in a number of ways. Scientific theories reflect ideological positions and values which are rarely explicitly stated. A prime example of this is the way that premenstrual syndrome is so often defined as a disability at times when women are wanted out of the workforce.[4] Bias also intrudes into decisions about what is studied and what is not. So, for example, the negative aspects of the menstrual cycle are studied and re-emphasised repeatedly, while few study the creativity women experience during the cycle. Men's hormonal cycles are rarely studied, to discover whether men are periodically 'unbalanced' and 'irrational'.

The ideology of science is intimately related to its historical development. As Galileo's and then Darwin's explanations of the world became accepted, science replaced religion as an authority. The emerging view of the new scientific age was 'masculinist', seeing women as alien and inexplicable. Ehrenreich and English write:

> Everything that seems uniquely female becomes a challenge to the rational scientific intellect. Woman's body, with its autonomous rhythms and generative possibilities, appears to the masculinist vision as a 'frontier', another part of the natural world to be explored and mined. A new science—Gynaecology—arose in the nineteenth century to study this strange territory and concluded that the female body is not only primitive, but deeply pathological.[5]

Ruth Bleier, a professor of neurophysiology and women's studies, has written a critique of biological theories about women which she claims amount to 'an elaborate mythology of women's biological inferiority as an explanation for their subordinate position in the cultures of Western civilisations'. Science, she says, has divided civilisation into contradictory and dichotomous spheres, male and female, and has developed 'a dualistic mode of thought, the development of concepts and ideologies of oppositions, dominance and subordinance, culture and nature, and subject and object'.[6] The scientific ethic, as Kathy Overfield has commented, like capitalism and imperialism, is 'based on exploitation, elimination of rivals, domination and oppression'.[7] Leaders of research in the reproductive area are deified as if they are 'acting God'. The danger of this deification is that both the medical profession and the community may feel that medical teams are not accountable to the society in which they work. The scientific mystique fosters the creation of experts to control our lives; masculine experts to replace the male God. A certain awe surrounds these men because of their 'control' of nature. The sometimes veiled (in the case of reproductive technology, articulated) threat exists that the knowledge they control may be withdrawn, leaving us with no 'progress'.

In order to 'progress' within the hierarchical and competitive structure of science, scientists must obtain grants for research and must publish. This can only be done if the area is suitable in the view of grant-givers, publishers and promotions committees. Institutions like the Rockefeller Foundation thus operate in a gatekeeping manner. Women scientists tend to find the scientific environment hostile. They comment on the undesirability of acquiring the necessary 'male' values needed for success. Here 'openness is anathema',

> emotional dishonesty is blatant under guises of reason, objectivity and abstractions, and where the social reasons for doing science are lost among the emotional needs of Western men to achieve, perform and acquire status in the eyes of their own sex.[8]

The so-called ability of males to isolate one aspect and to narrowly pursue it, which is said to be necessary for the successful scientist, leads to a tunnel vision which limits scientific foresight to the laboratory, mitigates against it being honest and accountable within broader social structures and makes it difficult to apply scientific findings to a world where in reality all things are connected. Over and over we ask why people starve, why women cannot have a safe contraceptive, why breast cancer is still a killer —while men put themselves on the moon or into orbit, thus symbolically distancing themselves from the concerns of Earth.

THE STRUGGLE FOR CONTROL OVER REPRODUCTION

As science developed its ethic of understanding and then dominating nature, it constructed its rationale for the control of woman, particularly as she represented the forces of nature in reproduction. Francis Bacon had called on men to turn their 'united forces against the Nature of things, to storm and occupy her castles and strongholds'. He urged them 'to bind [Nature] to your service and make her your slave'.[9]

The suppression of women healers and midwives culminated in the witch-burnings in Europe. The emergence of male midwives in the seventeenth century marked the beginning of the so-called management of childbirth.[10] It is symbolically marked by the invention of obstetric forceps by the men of the Chamberlen family who kept them secret for three generations, using the forceps under a sheet so that no one could observe their actions and they could maintain their monopoly.[11]

The fact was that male midwives had little understanding of the processes of labour and childbirth. Yet male control of birth was institutionalised in the development of the first lying-in hospital in London in 1739. As Anna Macgarvey rightly points out, these hospitals achieved

> not only the opportunity for men-midwives to gain clinical experience, but also the restriction of competition from female practitioners, the establishment of control over patient preferences and the definition of childbirth as a hazardous event without the attendance by the men-midwives.[12]

The unfortunate result of this hospitalisation of women was an epidemic of puerperal or childbed fever, which killed many women.[13] Though in 1861 a Viennese physician, Semmelweis, had made the connection between the practices of men midwives and puerperal fever, showing how it could be avoided by more care and simple hygiene precautions, male midwives continued to blame women themselves.

> The reluctance of men-midwives and doctors to... adopt proper methods of cleanliness meant that puerperal fever continued to be the greatest single cause of maternal death through the nineteenth and into the twentieth century'.[14]

By the beginning of the nineteenth century, childbirth had changed from being a human experience to being a medical problem. Women mostly do not understand or know the processes of their own bodies; medicine has convinced them that they need help in order to get through childbirth—hence women go to a hospital (a place for sick people) when they are delivering.

In one textbook on pregnancy, *The Active Management of Labour*, the joint authors devote five paragraphs to the role of the mother in labour 'as distinct from her uterus, to which she is otherwise reduced'. The author of another of these popular books, *Pregnancy* (published initially in 1972 and in several later editions), cautions women not to turn to one another for advice. British obstetrician Gordon Bourne asserts that 'Probably more is done by wicked women with their malicious lying tongues to harm the confidence and happiness of pregnant women than by any other single factor'.[15] And his claim for the best source of advice? 'The final authority on any individual pregnancy is of course the doctor.'

The medical profession sees women's bodies as inefficient or defective. They are portrayed as machines in need of mechanics (doctors), and since they are prone to mechanical breakdown women have been increasingly subjected to technologised and impersonal forms of medical intervention which will control their pregnancy and birth experiences for them, and now indeed their conception experiences. It is a rare woman who manages her own pregnancy, labour and birth without any ultrasound, induction, fetal monitoring, amniocentesis, forceps delivery or caesarean section.

Not only is the woman's body defective but it is also a dangerous place for the embryo/fetus. For example, discussing the pregnancy rates using PROST (Pro Nuclear Stage Tubal Transfer), Dr John Yovich is quoted as saying that 'the results of PROST raised the possibility that the uterus was actually a hostile environment for the early embryo before a certain stage'.[16] Although it is the reproductive technology which fails women, they are still seen as the primary problem in the equation, just as male midwives continued to blame them for developing puerperal fever. One woman on an IVF programme said that when her ultrasound indicated that she was not producing enough follicles (eggs) to be harvested following superovulation using hormonal cocktails, the nurse said: '"Is that all there is? Come on Carol, you've gotta get them bigger"'. What did she think? 'Of course, I would like to make them as big as possible!'[17]

After fetal monitoring, ultrasound and induction of labour, the ultimate control for the doctor is of course a caesarean, but women often experience it as an assault, even a kind of rape. The statistics indicate that it is often questionable whether it is needed, and that its use depends on class and race: 'when there are clear clinical indications of fetal and maternal danger... more white women get a caesarean section, but when the labour is long or the rate of progression is slow, more black women get them'.[18] The caesarean rate in the US rose from 5 per cent in the late 1960s to 30 per cent in 1983. In Australia, by 1986 the rate of caesarean section had increased 300 per cent over the past two decades to 23 per cent. Of those giving birth vaginally, 81 per cent had episiotomy (an incision to enlarge the vaginal opening) and 48 per cent had a forceps delivery. No improvement in perinatal mortality resulted. In one study private patients had a higher rate of caesarean section and their babies had lower Apgar (birth health) scores.[19] Even caesarean section carried out because the fetus is in a breech presentation may be overused. In New York City Hospital during the 1970s there was an increase in the proportion of caesarean deliveries from 25 to 65 per cent with no change in the perinatal mortality rate of breech babies.[20]

Noting the high rate of the 'ritual sacrifice' of episiotomy, one British obstetrician said that the cut needed to be made because of potential damage which has been 'wrought by encouraging [women] to push too early and because the attendants are paying too much attention to the clock'. The time allowed for both the first and second stages of labour has been reduced steadily by the medical profession in Australia, the US and the UK since the 1940s: 'In short, the uterus... is being given less and less time to produce its product'.[21] The high use of forceps delivery is due to the widespread use of epidural anaesthesia 'which prolongs second stage of labour and renders it less efficient'.[22]

Doctors in the US are beginning to question the high incidence of caesarean section. At a conference sponsored by the Columbia University College of Physicians and Surgeons in 1987, Dr Friedman of Boston estimated that 50–70 per cent of caesarean sections are not necessary; the use of forceps could be avoided, he said, 'by simply monitoring the mother and fetus and waiting'. Many others at the conference agreed. Dr Gant, a professor of obstetrics and gynaecology at the University of Texas, also suggested that a financial incentive encouraged doctors to carry out caesareans unnecessarily.[23]

The issues of timing and control go hand in hand. Obstetricians in England treat with horror the suggestion that babies are induced 'for the convenience of themselves and their staff'; nevertheless, the figures indicate that babies 'generally prefer to be born on Thursdays and Fridays'! Thursday was the most popular day for 'spontaneous birth', Friday was the busiest day for 'induced labour' (25 per cent above the average) and Sunday was a loser (48 per cent below the average). The number of 'elective' caesarean sections, i.e. those not performed in an emergency, was 43 per cent above the average on Friday and 62 per cent below the average on Sunday.[24] This attitude is carried over into IVF deliveries and the superovulation of women to 'schedule'. Doctors resent having to be available on the weekends and have developed a new 'flare-up protocol' which makes it possible to 'organise in-vitro fertilisation or gamete intrafallopian transfers so that oocyte retrieval needs to be performed only rarely on Saturday and never on Sunday'.[25]

In her battle to allow women the birth of their choice and to avoid caesarean section, English doctor Wendy Savage became well known after her suspension from medical practice in April 1985 for allegedly allowing her patients to be endangered. Centring on five of the thousands of births for which she was a consultant obstetrician, the resulting enquiry made it quite clear that the issue was about medical power and practice. In her conclusion, Savage attacks thc increased medicalisation of birth and the elimination of midwives. She emphasises that

> this major change in childbirth patterns in society has been followed by increased medicalisation of birth and rising rates of intervention, without good scientific evidence that these high rates are necessary.[26]

Pryke et al. echo this in their Australian study:

> There seems reason to believe that new techniques have been introduced in obstetrics without scientific evaluation of outcomes. Instead of using new information and tools to identify women in need of special care, most women have been treated as being at risk.[27]

Medical intervention in childbirth is not only ineffective; it may be positively dangerous. For example in England and Wales 'both direct and indirect death rates are about ten times higher when delivery is by caesarean section rather than vaginal'.[28] As Dr Dermot McDonald of the National Maternity Hospital in Dublin, Ireland, commented,

> If one went to the extreme of giving the patient the full details of mortality and morbidity related to caesarean section, most of them would get up and go out and have their baby under a tree.[29]

Women have become more and more aware of the dangers of these interventions and their resistance is increasing. Martin documented incidents of resistance to caesarean section, induction, fetal monitoring and other technologies employed during birth. There is a real sense of joy from the woman who made it alone and who in the terms of her own doctor 'escaped' caesarean section. Martin writes that

> many women report simply unstrapping external fetal monitors the minute the nurse or doctor is out of the labour room. Others go for long walks around the hospital and do not return for hours or take a shower continuously so that monitors cannot be used.

She relates the story of the woman who was determined not to have a caesarean section for her second child, but who knew this would be the inevitable outcome because the baby was face up instead of face down as labour began. She actually used external massage to turn the baby and said: 'I didn't force her [the baby], I talked with her very carefully in what I was doing. I really worked with her'. By the time the ambulance had taken her to the hospital, the baby had turned all the way around and was born a few minutes after arrival.[30]

Such resistance may be more difficult in future, however, as the technology becomes more and more complex.

THE FRAGMENTATION AND DISMEMBERMENT OF WOMEN

Another characteristic of the development of medicine has been the separation of mind and body. Science treats a person as body only, divorced from feeling and thinking. This attitude makes the exchanging of body parts from person to person easier. Martin comments that

> the body as a machine without a mind or soul has become almost familiar, but the body without the integrity of even its parts will necessarily lead to many readjustments in our conceptions of the self, and the shape that will emerge is far from clear.[31]

In reproductive technology, women are described as 'uterine environments', wombs for rent. Ova which can be used in other women or turned into embryos for use in other women become exchangeable body parts. Medicine represents the carving up of women's bodies in its own divisions: obstetrics, gynaecology, paediatrics, neonatal paediatrics, fetal medicine, reproductive medicine, have symbolically segmented women's bodies for medical purposes.[32] In fetal medicine, the fetus becomes more and more the patient and an adversarial position is established by the medical profession between the woman and the fetus, particularly in the last trimester of pregnancy.

> Fetal medicine is also, significantly, the obstetrician's answer to the paediatrician's colonization of the immediate post-birth period with the subspeciality of neonatal paediatrics. Whether inside its mother's womb or not, the fetus-neonate is the subject of intra-professional rivalry. The moment of birth has become a line in a demarcation dispute.[33]

This fragmentation of women into body parts and interchangeable organs and cells is consonant with a tradition of constant experimentation on, and mutilation of, woman. If this seems too strong a way of putting it, consider the evidence on unnecessary surgery on women. For example, the rates of hysterectomy in Australia are now so high that the Doctors' Reform Society has condemned it; Dr Cynthia Cook has estimated that in the US today a woman has only a fifty/fifty chance of keeping her uterus and that only 15–30 per cent of hysterectomies are necessary.

In the nineteenth century in England and America, genital mutilation was practised. Although one of the major medical practitioners of the day, William Acton, stated that 'the majority of women are not very much troubled with sexual feelings of any kind', some women were found to be plagued by a variety of indispositions which needed a surgical cure: masturbation, nymphomania, and rebelliousness of character could be cured by clitoridectomy, and a range of disorders—troublesomeness, overeating, erotic tendencies, persecution mania—could be cured by ovariotomy (or female castration). Clitoridectomy was the first operation created in Western countries to control women's mental disorders. Middle- and upper-class women were usually the victims of these medical atrocities: their husbands could afford to pay for the 'treatment'. However, it was the poor and Black women who were guinea pigs for medical experimentation. In the US in the 1890s, pioneering gynaecological surgery was conducted by Dr Marion Sims 'on black female slaves he kept for the sole purpose of surgical experimentation'. On one of these women he performed thirty operations in four years. After he moved to New York, Sims used immigrant Irish women in the wards of the New York Women's Hospital as experimental subjects.[34]

Examples of the mutilation of women continue to surface in, for example, the work of American Dr James Burt who carried out 'love surgery' from 1966. He believed that the female anatomical system is faulty because women do not orgasm during penile penetration; therefore he surgically reconstructed the vagina and genitalia, dragging the clitoris closer to the vagina. When Burt wrote his book in 1975, four thousand women had been 'treated' by him, many without informed consent. Many of these had had their bodies 'redesigned' following birth when they thought they had had episiotomy and repair. As Janet Phillips, who went to Burt for cramps and ended up 'redesigned', said: 'You're raised to trust your minister, your policeman and your doctor. He was the one with the degree on the wall. He knew medicine better than I did. I didn't think he would hurt me.'[35] In his book Burt wrote that 'women are structurally inadequate for intercourse. This is a pathological condition amenable to surgery... the difference between rape and rapture is salesmanship'. Medical colleagues watched silently for twenty-two years while Burt performed his mutilations, before the Ohio State Medical Board charged him with 'gross immorality' and 'grossly unprofessional conduct'.

Gena Corea documents cases of women who have had surgery done to them without their permission, often under the label 'biopsy'. In one instance nurses at a hospital in Ohio 'mentioned that three physicians routinely performed clitoridectomies on all their patients who delivered babies in that hospital'. The nurses were relieved when Blue Cross/

Blue Shield medical insurance ceased to reimburse for clitoridectomies. Corea also lists incidences of the deliberate mutilation of women who went in for a biopsy only to have a vulvectomy, involving the removal of the inner labia. Needless to say these particular operations all negatively affect the woman's sexual pleasure.[36]

The assumption that medicine is universally benign is dangerously misleading. Although true healing is the concern of many general practitioners, there are also many doctors involved in the torture of people under various repressive regimes throughout the world, as Amnesty International has pointed out. In so-called democratic free societies such as the United States experimentation has been conducted on prisoners for many years. Dr Ewen Cameron, a highly regarded doctor in Britain, Canada and the US and titled the 'godfather' of Canadian psychiatry, became involved with the CIA and used his patients as subjects in experimental psychiatric and psychological work. Ironically, Dr Cameron was in Nuremberg to help write the code of ethics for medical experiments after the horrors of the Nazi doctors' work in World War II. 'The code to which he contributed—but did not adopt—stipulated that patients should be informed and given the right to consent to medical experiments.'[37]

Women are repeatedly used as testing populations for new drugs, and this continues with the testing of hormones on 'captive' populations of IVF women. But they are also used in clinical trials in which the Nuremberg Code is a dead letter. In 1988 and 1989 there was a public scandal in New Zealand over the 'unfortunate experiments' carried out on women attending the National Women's Hospital for suspected or confirmed cancer. Herbert Green, an international expert on cervical cancer at the hospital, saw between 1956 and 1982 some 1800 women with the potential early stages of cervical cancer. His theory was that indications of abnormal cell development would not necessarily lead to invasive cancer, though others in the profession held the view that if a smear from the cervix revealed cell changes in the earlier stages, they should be treated as cancerous. But as Sandra Coney and Phillida Bunkle, who uncovered the scandal, wrote,

> This was never the intention of the National Women's experiment. Some women with evidence of disease were to be left. They would be followed—that is, brought back for regular smears and possibly more biopsies—but there was no intention to cure them.[38]

So women unknowingly could be harbouring an advanced stage of the disease and might even die. Green intended to observe the 'natural history' of the disease and to prove his thesis that untreated CIS (carcinoma in situ) did not lead to invasion of cancer. In the process he allowed women to go untreated and some of them died.[39]

Like many medical researchers/practitioners, Herbert Green did not think the patient should be the one who decided her treatment. He said, 'If we are uncertain about the natural history of the disease which cytology has revealed in [the patient], how can we possibly expect her to make what is really our decision?'[40] Chillingly, Coney and Bunkle could never get an assurance from the hospital that the experiment had ended. 'It was never formally stopped. No instructions were issued [by the hospital ethics committee] to doctors to abandon practices which by now had been shown to be dangerous'. Professor Dennis Bonham, head of the postgraduate school, said the study 'merged into general treatment. It stopped being a study and became general treatment'.[41] Once again experimentation becomes treatment or therapy.

Reproductive technology concerns itself with the control and manipulation of women's bodies; it is based on an ideological assumption that woman equals (inefficient) nature and that male medicine can do better. It constantly fragments and dismembers women during this process, and it uses women as experimental subjects, without obtaining their educated consent.

MEDICINE, SCIENCE AND COMMERCE

The rise of capitalism and the development of technology, medicine and science have been intimately connected. These interdependent structures affect the nature of health care which people receive, the level of risk which certain procedures and drugs entail, and the quality of healing available. It can be argued, for example, that because of the huge financial investment by companies in the production of fertility drugs and because of the need of medical researchers to 'harvest' more eggs from women for experimentation, neither can afford to stop producing/using these drugs and both may be blinded to the risks for women.

As I indicated in Chapter 2, genetic engineering companies are developing at a rapid rate and on an international scale. In an analysis of the genetic engineering companies and their products in the US, the *New York Times Business Day* indicated that 'the commercial payoff from genetic engineering is finally within sight'. Ronald Cape of the Cetus Corporation, a leading biotechnology company, predicted an 'avalanche in the next two years'.[42] One of the main concerns is the development of patents, which the companies indicate are vital to ensure a good financial return on what could be considered a risky investment. Some companies are making profits from selling laboratory instruments to other technology companies; some of them are involved in the development of plants resistant to herbicides; and others are concerned with the genetic engineering of drugs and vaccines for animals and then with the genetic engineering of animals themselves. The decision in the US in 1987 to allow the patenting of animals was a major step. Randall Charlton, president and chief executive of University Genetics, which is involved in work producing leaner beef and cows with greater milk yield, said, 'It would allow us to put the UGen brand on a new supercow and nobody would be able to rustle it'. The two main breeders of chickens in the United States, Arbor Acres Farm Inc. and Hubbard Farms, a division of a pharmaceutical giant, Merck and Company, are developing chickens that grow faster on less feed.[43] Large profits are also expected to come from the genetic engineering of pharmaceuticals, including human insulin and human growth hormone. There were four genetically engineered pharmaceuticals on the market in 1987 which brought $150 million in sales. In 1987 biotechnology companies grossed more than $679 million from public stock offerings, 100 times the amount in the previous year.[44]

Biomedical technology alone is developing a huge market. In the US, Silicon Valley has been followed by Bionic Valley, developed by the University of Utah among others. The university takes equity in the companies using its research in what it calls 'academic capitalism', a 'marrying' of medicine and engineering. This has resulted in such developments as an artificial heart and, foreseeably, artificial blood vessels, heart valves, urinary sphincters and fallopian tubes.[45]

James Twerdahl, Marketing Director of Fertility and Genetics Research Company has said that 'infertility is a huge market'. It is estimated that in their desire for children, couples in the US will spend between $400 million and $500 million each year. In 1987, Serono Laboratories Inc. was the sole American supplier of Pergonal, a drug used in infertility treatment: its sales in 1982 were $7.2 million, but by 1986 they had risen to $35 million. As Sandra Blakeslee comments, 'the estimated $30 million to $40 million market in IVF procedures has medical entrepreneurs interested, especially since insurers are starting to pick up some of the costs'.[46]

The development of surgical instruments for the new techniques is also fertile financially, if not in terms of producing children. A special probe developed and sold by the Genetics and IVF Institute in Fairfax cost $120 000. The manufacturer of medical equipment from Diasonics Inc. in California, Bill Carrano, estimates that special probes and ultrasound equipment are likely to raise nearly $35 million in the next few years.[47] Fertility and Genetics Research Inc., a Chicago company, was awarded a patent on instruments to harvest fertilised eggs, and then applied for a patent on the entire medical procedure of embryo flushing. This particular company has entered into a franchising arrangement with groups of doctors in California and has estimated that eventually IVF could be a $6 billion annual business; though as Blakeslee pointedly comments, 'For now, though, IVF clinics will have to learn how to make more babies before they can make more money'.[48]

The infertile have been discussed as 'the ever-growing market'. Dr John Kerin of the University of Adelaide's Queen Elizabeth Hospital said before he left to take up a new position in the US that 'the demand is enormous and we are not competing with other groups for couples. The workload is very very heavy. There is more than enough for everyone'.[49] Bob Moses, chairman of the board of IVF Australia (in Australia and the USA), was said to be setting his sights on a $19 billion market from the 'three million baby-starved couples in the United States who want children but are unlikely to have them except by so-called heroic means, such as in-vitro fertilisation'.[50]

IVF Australia was the first company in Australia to establish itself, in March 1985, amid fierce public debate. The intention was to make profit through selling the know-how and expertise of the Monash University IVF team, particularly in the area of cryo-preservation (the freezing of embryos and the intended freezing of eggs), and hormonal stimulation of ovulation.[51] The proposal for this company was first presented to the Council of Monash University, a government-funded institution, in November 1984. A member of the university council then leaked the proposal to the press and it caused a very strong public response. The initial plan from the finance committee to council was intended for approval not debate, and included the stipulation that Monash University would have an equity in the company. Members of the council were not told the names of the backers or the directors of the company and were not given details of the actual proposal.

In the final arrangements, Monash agreed to a 300 per cent royalty arrangement but did not allow direct shareholding on the part of its academic staff. In 1985 Monash was paid an advance of \$200 000–\$300 000 to expand its obstetrics and gynaecology facilities. Future royalties were to help fund in vitro fertilisation research. The *Monash Review* noted test-tube babies as one of the 'range of inventions which Monash has become involved in selling over the years'.[52]

Although IVF Australia established clinics in New York State and Alabama in the US it was also looking at the possibility of establishing clinics in Singapore, Japan and other countries. The profit forecast was \$6.5 million (Australian) for each clinic per year in revenue when fully operational. As Bob Moses (then Director) commented:

> We are different from the other US programs, which have links with the universities and have problems sorting

> out the priorities between their research and commercial objectives. *Our objective is totally commercial* (my emphasis).[53]

In March 1988, dissatisfied with IVF Australia, Monash University set up a further private company, Infertility Medical Centre Pty Ltd, naming as shareholders Monash University, Dr Carl Wood and Dr Alan Trounson. The company's secretary and general manager, David Hodge, said the company did not intend to market the centre's techniques but was intended to ensure that money made from the medical centre at the Epworth Hospital went to the Centre for Early Human Development at Monash University of which Dr Trounson was the director. This centre was doing research into micro-injection techniques and work on early embryos. Other money would go to the Department of Obstetrics and Gynaecology at the university.[54]

A third Australian company is PIVET, standing for Programmed In Vitro Fertilisation and Embryo Transfer. This company was established in Perth as a public company to 'tap potential multi-billion-dollar untouched markets in Britain, Europe, Asia, North Africa and the Middle East'. It intended to sell scientific know-how, equipment and computer software developed by a privately run research team. From a modest beginning, relying on 'funds raised through lamington drives and the sale of home-made jams and cakes by a loyal and dedicated band of childless wives and would-be grandmothers', Pivet Australia developed into a $5 million complex with a team of scientists and technicians of international renown. In 1985 Pivet established a laboratory in Pantai, Malaysia, and later it set up similar complexes in Kuala Lumpur and Athens; other laboratories were planned for Hong Kong, Naples, Singapore, Cairo and Britain. The chairman of Pivet, Terry Miles, indicated that infertility treatment and the equipment associated with infertility treatment had become 'a lucrative export commodity'. Their computer software 'provides the data for a whole range of complex decisions which have to be made each day with each patient undergoing treatment'. The intention of this technology was to 'bypass a decade of fumbling around trying to achieve a successful pregnancy'.[55] Once again this means a lack of concern for individual women. In this delicate intrusion into women's bodies individual treatment, not standardised, computerised assessment, is needed. Ignoring the eugenics policy of the government in Singapore, though admitting that it discourages the breeding of children by those from other than professional backgrounds, Miles said: 'When you consider that about 15 per cent of the population in most developed countries is infertile, the prospective clientele is enormous... Malaysia alone has a population of 14 million'.[56]

Australian doctors have become particularly entrepreneurial, marrying IVF treatment with the Asian tourist trade to Australia. Allamanda Private Hospital on the Gold Coast, assisted by Professor Carl Wood, was offering tourist packages in 1989 to Japanese, Filipino and Singaporean couples. In Sydney, a private clinic was offering a similar package. 'It's a form of assisting the tourist industry', said the director, Dr John Anderson. 'What could be more natural [*sic*] than to go for a month's holiday and when you come back, be pregnant'.[57]

The basic premise on which all of this money-making is founded is that there will be a continuing infertile population: indeed 'to be profitable, IVF clinics must generate high patient volume to cover the extremely high fixed and operating costs associated with IVF'.[58] Science cannot afford to cure infertility. As Dr Sher of the Nevada Clinic said, 'The whole thing in IVF is numbers. You need to go above a certain threshold to make a lot of money'.[59]

THE DANGERS OF COMMERCIALISATION

The concern generated in the Australian community when IVF Australia was established is not unique. Academics are also worried about Bionic Valley in the US, pointing to the possibility of conflict of interest arising from personal profit, and of research monies being directed to one particular area of research while other areas are neglected. Some universities in the US have drawn up guidelines about outside work. Early in 1982 the State of California's Fair Political Practices Commission (FPPC) decided that academic freedom was not a sufficient defence for the non-disclosure of commercial interests: 'they adopted a recommendation that all university faculty members should be required to divulge their financial interests in any company sponsoring their work at the university'. A further possible conflict is raised in guidelines at Harvard which now state explicitly that potential conflict could be generated if a member of the faculty 'directs students into a research area from which a member hopes to realise financial gain'. In the case of the Bionic Valley, Raymond White, co-chairman of the Human Genetics Department at Utah, has expressed his concern that graduate students could 'become low-paid lackeys of the company'. He points out that the student may have the 'pleasure of seeing his work become public domain but the faculty member has the pleasure of taking it to the bank'.[60] There is also the possible filching of work by a scientist for the benefit of the company. For example, in reviewing research grant applications, scientists may garner information which can be used for their own purposes within a commercial enterprise.

Also of concern is the concept of freedom of information, particularly about research in publicly funded institutions such as Australian universities. The public pays for this work through the funding of the institution and also through taxes paid to government which are given out as research grants. Resulting research material should be available for public discussion. This is particularly true in the area of infertility, where the research is supposedly undertaken to help the infertile, yet commercial enterprises are unlikely to allow free publication of information in scientific journals until their commercial control and profit are ensured. Any premature disclosure can mean the rejection of the patent application, so 'the most prudent course is to say and publish nothing until the provision specification is publicly available eighteen months after being filed'.[61]

Sheldon Krimsky, a former member of the Recombinant DNA Advisory Committee to the National Institutes of Health in the US, is concerned that the more academic scientists become financially involved with industry, the more they may ignore the social impact of their work. He suggests that

> values, which emphasize science for commerce, will most likely become internalised and rationalised as a public good. A transformation of the disciplinary conscience can take place. These changes can happen incrementally and without malice. Scientists/engineers with a stake in the commercial outcome of a field cannot, at the same time, retain a public interest perspective that gives critical attention to the perversion of science in the interests of markets.[62]

The relationship between medical research and commerce opens up possibilities for the misuse of the results of scientific research. One case concerned the work of Professor Michael Briggs, a research scientist at Deakin University in Victoria who alledgedly 'falsified research on the effects of the low-dose contraceptive pills, Logynon and Trinordiol'. Professor Briggs published his work in major journals such as the *Lancet* and the *British Medical Journal* and was a consultant for the World Health Organisation. His name appeared in the advertisement for Logynon by Schering. There is no wrong-dealing on the part of the commercial company involved, but there is a misleading air of scientific objectivity attached to work which is essentially commercial. Briggs' research was published in the reputable *Journal of Reproductive Medicine* in a supplement which was financed by Schering.

> Schering, acting quite honestly and openly, paid for the professor's research, paid for the conference, paid for the proceedings to be published in that supplement, and provided offprints for doctors.

Veitch has commented:

> There is widespread agreement within the profession that doctors have come to rely far too heavily on drug money. The 'inducements', as the college [Royal College of Physicians] puts it, are threatening patients' safety and the integrity of the profession.[63]

The most important concern, however, is that when medical research is so heavily involved in and dependent on drugs and saleable technologies/techniques, it will not focus on preventative medicine.

THE ROLE OF THE STATE

Increasingly the state is drawn into the inter-relationship between commerce and medicine. Dr Cape of Cetus Biotechnology Company in the US indicates that 'the biotechnology industry rests on a foundation of $100 billion in federal spending on basic health science research over the last forty years'. Company executives are indicating that the threat to increased commercial profits in the US comes from a possibility of cutbacks in federal spending on health research.[64] Australian scientists constantly bemoan what they consider to be a lack of government spending in the medical research area, and repeatedly threaten to leave the country because of the lack of encouragement to commercial enterprise: 'research units across Australia were crying out for funds and struggling to stop their most brilliant scientists from moving overseas'.[65]

Yet the community which pays taxes for research funding could more validly argue that low-tech solutions to problems of infertility and research into the causes of infertility are totally ignored by the federal government. In Australia, the Department of Industry, Technology and Commerce in its Biotechnology Grants Scheme for 1989-91 stated as its aim an encouragement of collaboration between industry and research groups in academic institutions, highlighting genetic engineering, biotechnology, and human pharmaceutical/medical research as top priorities. In 1988, of the $37 million dispensed by the Medical Research Endowment Fund of the National Health and Medical Research Council, $1.84 million went to genetic engineering and genetically related research; community health research was allocated about $160 805. IVF-related research received $433 659 while no money was given to research into the prevention of infertility. Breast cancer, the single biggest cause of death in Australian women, received $42 923 in research funds and cervical cancer $232 131, when each year about 340 women die of cervical cancer, while another 1000 cases are discovered when they are so advanced that they must be treated by removing the uterus and often the ovaries and the fallopian tubes.[66]

State governments too are encouraging technological developments which might prove profitable. For example, the Victorian state government had a stake in IVF Australia, through its Victorian Economic Development Corporation. The Minister for Industry, Technology and Resources rejected a suggestion that this represented a conflict of interests,[67] although the government had established a committee under its Infertility (Medical) Procedures Act to oversee and control embryo experimentation. This conflict of interest can also be seen in the presence of a Health Department representative on the board of Infertility Medical Centre Pty Ltd in Melbourne.

A disturbing statement in a paper on IVF Australia by the Vice-Chancellor of Monash University, Professor Ray Martin, in 1987, indicated a close connection between university and government which could have precluded an independent government position on embryo experimentation. Martin writes:

> It has been particularly satisfying that the Government of Victoria through its Minister for Health has regarded the Monash Ethics Committee, which was established originally for the purposes of the agreement with IVF Australia Pty Ltd, as an important source of advice on ethical issues raised in the wider debate in the community.[68]

Fortunately, the government did resist an approach from Monash University to have the Freedom of Information Act changed in order to protect its potential commercial interests. Monash, on behalf of the four Victorian universities, requested the Attorney-General to amend the legislation to protect information about research even before work had started, for example research projects which were in a proposal form and made in grant applications.[69] This would have made it more difficult for the public to find out about experimentation undertaken by reproductive technology teams.

SCIENTIFIC ACCOUNTABILITY

The state of Victoria provides a textbook study of the relationship between medical research scientists, the state, commercial enterprises and the law. The legislation which was established in Victoria in 1985, the Infertility (Medical) Procedures Act, banned embryo experimentation. Under considerable pressure from doctors the state government decided to change the law to allow experimentation on embryos up to twenty-two hours or syngamy (when the nuclei of the egg and sperm fuse).

In some instances the conduct of researchers seems to indicate an unwillingness to carry out the intention of legislation which is in the process of being drawn up or proclaimed. For example, doctors may move patients to avoid ethics committees. In 1983 the Monash University team, led by Dr Alan Trounson and Professor Carl Wood, had an ovum donor programme at the Queen Victoria Medical Centre. While agreeing to a moratorium at this public hospital, as requested by the state Premier and acting Attorney-General, John Cain, the team did what Professor Carl Wood said could be called 'a smart switch' in continuing to carry out the procedure at the Epworth Hospital which had *not* been approached by the Premier on this issue.[70]

In April 1988 scientists flaunted the spirit, if not the reality, of impending legislation. Research scientists had argued quite strongly that the law needed to be changed, principally to allow them to do experiments with micro-injection of sperm. It was later revealed that this very experiment had been done and the embryos implanted into women, without checking them for abnormalities. This was possible because the legislation is concerned about protecting the embryo but has no concern with protecting the women involved. The women were to be used as living laboratories to see whether the embryo would be normal or not. As one scientist said, 'they were really going through a bit of a clinical trial. In some ways, I suppose, each patient is sort of experimental'.[71] Once again scientists seem unable to accept that they are accountable to the society in which they live and work and on whom their research has such a major impact.

Within this continuing battle, one of the most common threats is that the research team will leave the country. In 1983, Dr Alan Trounson threatened to withdraw from the IVF programmes unless reasons were given for the moratorium on donor ova work.[72] In 1986, Dr Trounson was still issuing ultimatums that he and his team would go overseas within six months if they were not allowed to continue research on embryos.[73] In 1988, he was once again threatening to take the research team overseas if the legislation was not hurriedly proclaimed in order to allow micro-injection work. He pointed out that salaries were much higher overseas and they could get on with their research there.[74]

In 1986 Dr John Kerin followed through on such a threat and took his whole medical research team from the University of Adelaide's Queen Elizabeth Hospital to the Jones Centre in Norfolk, Virginia, which had received a $28 million grant from the American government for infertility research. It was the 'unlimited resources' which lured them. In 1986 Dr Hugh Niall, who had previously worked at the Howard Florey Institute in Melbourne determining the structure of the hormone Relaxin, also went to the US to become Director of Research and Developmental Biology with the San Francisco-based biotechnology company, Genentech. He pointed out that again the research budget had lured him and that in the company everybody worked extremely long hours and at weekends. He said: 'Generally, the ethic is to get the work done in the knowledge that it's a highly competitive situation and the success of the company depends on everyone's efforts'.[75] Genentech shares can be bought by employees at reduced costs, so researchers benefit from company profits.

Similar behaviour occurs in genetic engineering when legislation threatens research and commerce. Glick reports on a company that extracts growth hormone and has a subsidiary involved in genetic engineering: 'It has been reported that the Swedish subsidiary may have to leave Sweden because of the severe restrictions there pertaining to recombinant DNA research'.[76]

What these continuing threats amount to is the refusal of scientists to be socially accountable for their work and the inability of government to stand by decisions made after community debate when pressure is applied from commercial interests and the medical profession. Doctors promise that the medical profession will be self-regulating, but their behaviour does not encourage faith in this system: they lack ethical credibility. Where there is so much profit to be made, they cannot be the guardians of our ethical values. The lesson in Victoria to date is that the power bloc formed by medical research and commercial interests is a very strong challenge to the role of government in controlling research which intimately affects every person in our society. According to Dr Glick, President of Genex Corporation in the US,

> I do not know how to emphasise this too much, but it is the stock incentive that has really turned the scientists on. I think there is a lesson to be learned here.[77]

6. 'REPROSPEAK': THE LANGUAGE OF THE NEW REPRODUCTIVE TECHNOLOGIES

LANGUAGE SETS THE CONTEXT

Part of the strategy of social control which powerful groups use is the construction of a language which creates a 'softening up phase',[1] language which prepares people for ideas or technologies which would otherwise be unacceptable. Medical scientists are no novices in this area. Their language defines women as defective and reveals a desire for control over women and reproduction, alongside an unconscious dismembering of women into interchangeable body parts.

As I indicated in the earlier chapters, scientists can describe a birth mother as merely a substitute ('surrogate'); they can describe the surgical procedure of taking a fetus from a brain-dead woman as 'giving birth', implicitly normalising the procedure; and they can falsify failed technologies by discussing only 'success rates', rather than 'failure rates' when 92 per cent of clients go home without a child. The effect of such use of language is insidious and pervasive. It infiltrates media reporting of reproductive technology, influences the legal system so that judges see women as 'alternative reproduction vehicles', and convinces women themselves of their role as 'incubators'.[2]

Language and naming are very powerful in shaping the attitudes of a society. Reprospeak, the language of reproductive technology, has been used to convince people that these technologies are innocuous procedures developed to assist the infertile. Those people who do have children are made to feel guilty if they try to criticise or stand in the way of those 'infertile' people seeking assistance. The term 'infertile' has been used very loosely however. Women may be unable to conceive due to pelvic inflammatory disease; sexually transmitted diseases; the use of IUDs and other contraceptive devices; sterilisation during a prior marriage; poorly performed abdominal surgery or post-operative infection in anything from an appendix operation to an abortion (iatrogenic or doctor-induced infertility). As Dr Robert Winston, a leading IVF specialist at the Hammersmith Hospital in London, said,

> We found that nearly all [the women we treated] had marked adhesions or damage, often of extreme severity, which could be largely attributed to inappropriate tissue handling, avoidable post-operative infection, or removal of potentially viable organs.[3]

(Ironically, in some cases infertility treatment may have caused the problem. In one case a 'surrogate' was engaged to bear a child for a woman who was infertile because she had had problems in a pregnancy on an IVF programme in England, had lost the baby and had to have a hysterectomy.[4])

But 30 per cent of infertile couples are so defined because of male infertility, and a further third have the cause diagnosed as 'idiopathic'—basically, unknown. In Australia and New Zealand between 1979 and 1988, 7.5 per cent of couples were on the programme because of specific male-factor infertility, 25 per cent were on the programme because of multiple causes which would have included a male problem, and about 12 per cent were there for unexplained infertility. These figures are likely to increase considerably with greater use of micro-injection, a procedure used to alleviate male infertility; thus an increasing number of healthy women who are not themselves infertile will undergo potentially dangerous treatment. Women can also be using IVF for secondary infertility; they have one child but cannot conceive or carry a second child. In 1988, following the patterns of previous years, over half the clients for IVF and GIFT had had previous pregnancies.[5]

More and more women are being deemed 'infertile' by virtue of their husband's infertility. In a case of IVF surrogacy in Victoria, which occurred before it was illegal, the Solicitor-General declared that the fertile sister was deemed to be infertile by virtue of her own husband's vasectomy.[6] As mentioned in Chapter 4, many women in couples recruiting 'surrogate' mothers are or have been fertile: the wife of Patricia Foster's sperm donor had three children by a previous marrige, and the wife of Alejandra Munoz's sperm donor had a daughter by a previous marriage.

The language used often conflates the woman with the couple, so that a false picture is given that both parties experience the invasiveness of IVF. One medical centre in the US wrote that 'we are looking at the possibility of using host [surrogate] mothers to incubate embryos for couples with no or damaged uterus'.[7]

Researchers manipulate the language to reconstruct the reality of reproductive technology for the public. The construction of a 'pre-embryo' is a good example. This took place in Victoria in the debates in 1988 and 1989 on changing the law banning embryo experimentation, as well as in England where similar ploys were used. Scientists have argued that an embryo is only an embryo when the nuclei of the egg and the sperm fuse, about twenty-two hours after the egg has allowed the sperm to enter it. Hence the 'pre-embryo' was born! This character very soon became a 'fertilised egg'; it is more acceptable for scientists to fiddle with 'eggs' than to manipulate 'embryos'.

The pressures on women are hidden in the simplistic descriptions given to the public. It is simply said that an egg is taken from the woman, sperm from the man, an embryo is created and reimplanted in the woman. Yet the picture changes dramatically in women's descriptions of the procedure. In a number of hospitals, the woman is required to kneel on all fours to have the embryos inserted. There has never been a medical reason given for this process. One woman describes this degrading and pornographic procedure thus:

> Two days after surgery, I went back for the embryos to be transferred into my uterus. When they put them in with the fluid, I was scared to move. I had to stay on my hands and knees with my rear end elevated for the transfer—all of this with eight people looking at me. What a humiliating position.[8]

Many of the issues raised in the previous chapter on the relationship between medical science and women are reflected in the language of the new reproductive technologies: the picture of woman as Nature, most often defective and inefficient; the language of dismemberment and objectification; the related language of control or the desire to control both women and the reproductive process; and the language of commercialisation defining the child as a product. The language used by scientists and by the popular media which transmits their information to the public exemplify these constructions.

WOMAN AS NATURE, DEFECTIVE AND INEFFICIENT

Women are treated as animal nature by medical researchers. This allows them to distance themselves from the humanity of women and to ignore the emotional impact of their experimentation. A good example of this is the statement made by Australian doctors John McBain and Alan Trounson discussing the treatment of patients in in vitro fertilisation: 'the human female is capable of having substantial litters under certain circumstances...'. Women are described as fields to be 'harvested' for eggs, a doctor carrying out a laparoscopy is described as being 'like a miner panning for human gold'.[9] In her poem 'Right to Life' Marge Piercy, claiming the right of women to chose an abortion in a society which refuses to take care of all its children, writes:

> Now you legislate mineral rights in a woman.
> you lay claim to her pastures for grazing,
> fields for growing babies like iceberg lettuce.
> You value children so dearly,
> that none ever go hungry...
> ...Every noon the best
> restaurants serve poor children steaks.[10]

Though all human beings begin as female and need a shot of testosterone in the embryonic stage in order to develop into a male at around the seventh week—being what one journalist describes as 'sexually indifferent' [11]—woman is still represented as an absence. Christopher Joyce writes of science having discovered the genetic switch which determines sex and notes that 'if it is absent, the fetus develops into a female'.[12]

This language of absence applied to the developing fetus marks the beginning of the definition of woman as defective or inefficient, particularly in labour and birth as was shown in Chapter 5. According to Dr Gary Hodgen, scientific director of the Howard and Georgeanna Jones Institute for Reproductive Medicine in Norfolk, human reproduction is 'inherently inefficient even in normal, fertile couples'.[13] But it is not to the 'couples' that science turns its attention; it is to the woman.

In discussing ovulation and the development of ovarian cancer, Fathalla in the *Lancet* writes that

> Compared with other mammals, the human female appears to be very *extravagant* with her ova. Ovulatory cycles are almost continuous from puberty to the menopause. Other mammals are *more economical* with their ova (my emphasis).[14]

He continues that ovarian cancers relate to 'extravagant and mostly *purposeless* ovulation in the human female'.

In another example, Dr Gabor Kovacs and his colleagues discuss the multiple pregnancy rate following use of human pituitary gonadotrophin. The problem, according to scientists, does not lie in the drugs used to superovulate, it lies with the woman.

> The quintuplet pregnancy was the result of an atypical response. It is interesting that when the same patient received another course of treatment, it again resulted in an inappropriate response.[15]

An underlying anger at the woman's body for not performing as instructed repeatedly surfaces. An Australian government report describes some women as infertile because they have 'hostile or lethal uterine environments'.[16]

Emily Martin has analysed the language in medical texts describing menopause and menstruation. Menopause is described as a state in which the ovaries become 'unresponsive' or 'regress'. She writes: 'at every point in this system functions "fail" and falter. Follicles "fail to muster the strength" to reach ovulation'. One medical writer even describes the ovaries as 'senile'.[17] When science fails in its attempt to implant an embryo into the uterus, the embryo constructed by science along with science itself remains blameless. Discussing the research of Dr Peter Rogers at Monash University, Susan Downie writes:

> By growing rat embryos on the eyes of other rats, he has discovered that an embryo will implant itself in almost any tissue, and failure to implant is the fault of the uterus, not the embryo. This means that to improve the success rate IVF scientists should now concentrate on preparing the uterus to receive the embryos.[18]

The battle that takes place in scientific medicine to improve on the natural functioning of a woman's body takes some ironic turns, as in the technique described in Chapter 1, which

> allows the woman to be a human incubator for her own embryos. Instead of the eggs and sperm being placed in culture in a petri-dish and spending their first 48 hours in a laboratory incubator, they (and the culture) go into a tiny tube that is put into the woman's vagina, held in place by a diaphragm.[19]

A second 'back to nature' technique is described as a new culture in which to assist the egg and the embryo to fertilise in vitro; the culture turns out to be 'simple amniotic fluid... so simple and so natural, you wonder why someone didn't try it earlier'.[20]

THE LANGUAGE OF DISMEMBERMENT, OBJECTIFICATION AND CONTROL

The language of dismemberment increases women's alienation from their bodies and from motherhood, signifying their loss of control of themselves as whole people. Body parts become interchangeable. Indeed, woman herself becomes merely a body part. In an article on the trade in human body parts, the list runs as follows: 'kidney $10 000, blood for hepatitis research $7500; fertile eggs [*sic*] $1500; sperm $55; surrogate motherhood [*sic*] $18 750'.[21]

Instead of discussing women as patients or as clients, doctors and scientists treat them as 'uterine environments', or in the words of one British specialist, 'endocrinological environments'.[22] In the Mary Beth Whitehead trial, Dr Lee Salk talked of women as 'surrogate uteruses' and in his judgement Judge Harvey Sorkow talked of women in surrogacy as 'alternative reproduction vehicles'. The American Fertility Society did likewise in its ethics report discussing the women as 'therapeutic modalities'.[23]

The linguistic dismembering of women's bodies into various interchangeable body parts—eggs, ovaries, wombs—is reflected in reality as science deals solely with the 'member at hand'; retranslating the woman's body part into a kind of laboratory. Hence the discussion above of the woman acting as an 'incubator' for her own embryo. Dr Gary Hodgen discusses the problems of embryo donation, seeing the solution in the storage of eggs before they are fertilised, creating what he terms an 'in-vitro ovary'.[24]

These conceptualisations of women are picked up by the popular press: a discussion of a new micro-injection technique in Melbourne failed to even use the word 'woman' in its discussion but said that the new technique was 'designed to make human embryos in the laboratory before transferring them to the womb'.[25] The women had become wombs only.

The alienation of women from their own bodies which this reinforces is particularly noticeable in the language used in discussions of surrogate motherhood. The woman is commonly represented as womb and capsule space, which can be easily bought or rented. The term 'surrogate mother' is itself a misnomer, as Chapter 4 points out. It is used to imply that the woman is somehow not the 'real' mother; yet the woman is in fact the birth mother. In order to make it easier for society to accept seeing a woman torn away from a child that she desires to keep, entrepreneurs in the surrogate industry and indeed scientists themselves have developed a variety of terms to describe this woman; she is the 'gestational mother', the 'host mother', the 'host womb' or as the Surrogate Parent Programme of Los Angeles named one of their surrogates, the 'Perfect Host'.[26]

Often the term 'mother' is not used at all. Women who give birth using another woman's egg are described as 'surrogate gestational carriers' or just 'gestational carriers'.[27] In its report on surrogacy, the Australian National Bioethics Consultative Council successfully depersonalised and disenfranchised birth mothers, describing them only as willing to 'gestate an embryo' or 'carry the child', as if there is no physical, emotional and psychological relationship between a woman and her developing fetus. The logical result of these word games is that the committee developed something it chose to call 'total surrogacy' where 'the surrogate mother has no genetic tie to the child other than that of being the agent of gestation', as opposed to 'partial' surrogacy when a birth mother uses her own genetic material. The intention is basically to deny birth mothers any status and to privilege a genetic donor. At the same time the fetus became personalised, exercising 'gestation of choice', an absurdity in a not yet living and independent being. The final linguistic absurdity was the creation of 'the surrogate child'.[28]

People who use a 'surrogate' mother as a way of having a child also use impersonal and mechanical language to convince themselves that they are not doing something which will damage the woman. An example is the infertile woman referred to in Chapter 4 who described her sister as a luggage container: 'We are just using Jacki as a suitcase really, an incubator to carry it. At the end of the day it is our child'.[29] Women themselves become accustomed to the dehumanisation of women and take upon themselves these objectifying self-definitions—like the Scottish woman already mentioned who described herself as a 'postie' just 'delivering the mail'.[30]

The surrogate industry defines women as 'for sale', and newspapers present this image to the public; 'in NSW, another couple is ready to buy the services of a woman's womb'. In the US, a company established by Harriet Blankfield, Miracle Program Inc., had 'twelve women on insemination stand-by'.[31]

The attack on motherhood itself is obvious. One reporter described the woman who receives a frozen embryo on IVF as an 'alien mother'.[32] And in his amazing construction of women as somehow not real mothers if they had babies outside marriage, ethicist John Robertson, noting the lack of babies for adoption now, put it down to the 'greater willingness of illegitimate mothers to keep their children'.[33] So while women's bodies are dismembered, women are also torn from their children symbolically and actually.

Scientists regularly assert that control is not their intention. Professor Carl Wood said: '... the motivation for our work came from women. There is no intention by us to control women'.[34] But medical scientists unintentionally reveal their desire to control the function of women's bodies through their language. Dr Alan Trounson writes that 'Edwards, Steptoe, Wood and his colleagues achieved IVF and initiated the vital first step of eliminating fertilisation from the restraints of body function'.[35] One doctor talked of a woman who had 'escaped' a caesarean section.[36]

Doctors discuss the uterus and the womb as an enemy, giving the impression that the womb is deliberately excluding them from its precincts. An Australian medico ponders whether a woman's system will continue to 'retain its present-day intra-uterine secrecy' and an American, apparently irritated with the necessity for medicine to accommodate to the rhythms of a woman's body, said: 'It means you have to be available at the right time: you have to be a prisoner of that woman's cervical mucus and her ovulation time'.[37]

Women's pregnancy is represented negatively, until and unless it is obvious/accessible to an 'outsider'. A journalist describes the experience of chorionic villus sampling (CVS) which is performed at nine to ten weeks of pregnancy:

> Because CVS can be performed at nine to ten weeks of pregnancy—*when the internal turmoil is sickeningly obvious to the woman but before its gentle external appearance is apparent to outsiders*—the technique offers a world of reassurance to parents worried about inherited diseases while giving the option of earlier, safe abortion, if necessary (my emphasis).[38]

Pregnancy is an illness, an enemy to be controlled and grappled with like a disease. A new 'contraceptive vaccine' would, it was claimed, 'immunise the body against pregnancy'.[39]

An odd corollary of the language of dismemberment which depersonalises women is the personalisation of body parts and gametes. Dr Ron Carson of Prince Henry's Hospital in Melbourne said that women having hysterectomy could be asked to donate slices of their ovaries for research, but that their ovaries might no longer be normal or useful: 'nubile young ovaries are very difficult to come up with: that's the problem'.[40] Eggs (ova) are talked of in the same way. According to Susan Downie, Dr Trounson seeks 'young eggs', because 'ova deteriorate in the body with age'. He does experiments on 'naked ova'.[41] As with surrogates, doctors like Dr Howard Jones look for a 'good egg' and even 'good sperm'.[42] Lasker and Borg even discuss the 'high mortality of fertilised eggs'.[43] Sperm, however, appear ageless!

But there is a dramatic difference in the language about eggs and sperm: though they may be able to have youth, age, and die, eggs do not have a 'mother' in the same way that sperm has a 'father'. Sperm is allocated child status. So for example in surrogacy, the man donating the sperm and buying the womb space of a woman is described as the 'father'. Likewise, in their discussion of AID Lasker and Borg write: 'There have in fact been a number of children who have tried to trace their fathers through medical school records or yearbooks'.[44] Sperm, not the parenting relationship, creates a 'father'.

Embryos are personalised in an extraordinary way. They can be 'orphaned', 'effectively parentless', or in their frozen state 'wait to find mothers'.[45] In a custody battle between divorcing partners over their frozen embryos, Judge Young in the US ruled that 'custody' should be awarded to the 'mother'. He ruled that they were not property, but children, 'human beings existing as embryos'.[46] As with eggs, scientists seek to grade embryos, preferring to implant 'high-calibre ones'. Embryos can also be 'wayward': Dr Melvyn Dodson is concerned that the low pregnancy rate on IVF is 'due in part to the tendency of embryos to fall out of the uterus immediately after placement'.[47]

Although doctors complain that groups campaigning against embryo experimentation turn the embryo into a person, they themselves commit this error constantly. Professor Bennett from the Sydney Royal Hospital for Women, discussing CVS which only takes place on a fetus nine to ten weeks old, said: 'That's one of the most exciting prospects in medicine—treating the unborn child'.[48]

Of course the embryo is also often given the ability to 'die'.[49] And just as the embryo became the 'pre-embryo' and then merely a 'fertilised egg' in order to avoid social constraints on embryo experimentation, a similar manipulation of terminology is used to make surrogate embryo transfer, a procedure in which an embryo is flushed from one woman and placed into another, acceptable. This has actually been referred to as 'prenatal adoption' and, more innocuously, 'ovum transfer'.[50]

Some doctors, on the other hand, talk of the embryo in technological terms as part of a commercial transaction. Dr John Buster, the originator of surrogate embryo transfer,

> described the embryo to us as a 'little microchip', a package containing an incredible amount of information. Now he is researching that package, decoding the information to discover defects in the chip.[51]

The fetus, as indicated in Chapter 3, is also personalised to the disadvantage of the woman. Described as 'he', it becomes a paramount 'patient' and 'seldom ever complains' and will 'at times need a physician'. 'He' resides in the 'dark inner sanctum' which becomes more and more 'transparent' with the use of technologies like ultrasound.[52] To treat this new patient may require 'aggressive fetal surgery'.[53] Aggressive to whom?

The language of control through ownership is also evident in the descriptions of doctors as the 'fathers of IVF'. After delivering the first baby born from the surgical extraction of sperm used with IVF, 'the two [doctors] were like excited new fathers at the weekend'.[54] When British doctor Ian Craft joined a celebratory get-together of test-tube children and mothers he was described as the 'daddy of them all', surveying his great 'family'. (It is notable that none of the biological fathers were in attendance or pictured in the photograph.) And 'fathers of IVF push the barriers further'. Carrying the desire for ownership of procreation into the concept of pregnancy itself, Dr John Yovich from Perth is described in the following way: 'He produced his first pregnancy in 1986'.[55] Likewise medical journalists constantly refer to the doctors' 'brainchild'. So the scientist becomes both the father of the living child, the father of the laboratory, the father of the idea, and of the scientific procedure.

COMMERCE AND THE NEW CHILD-PRODUCT

In Chapter 5 I showed the links between commercial interests and medical science, and this is apparent in the language used: 'Baby farming: the modern moral dilemma'.[56] The development of commercial reproductive technology has encouraged the perception of babies as a new 'product' to be marketed to the infertile. In discussing the development of PIVET (Programmed In-Vitro Fertilisation and Embryo Transfer), a company which was to be listed on the Perth Stock Exchange in order to raise a $4 million share issue, a news item said: 'Test-tube babies are about to hit the stock market'.[57]

The *New York Times* analysed the promotional efforts of IVF Australia in North America, discussing the hesitant response of the American market and other fertility clinics, using the language of the technology itself:

> But such promotional efforts meet with scepticism from some venture capitalists, who say fertility clinics probably can't be standardised and cloned into chains just yet, and therefore cannot generate enough volume to be sufficiently profitable.[58]

The development of reproductive technology companies and their relationship to investment is encapsulated in the title of a piece by Catherine Martin in the *Bulletin*: 'A new and fertile field for investment'. Elsewhere, it is described as a 'happy marriage of business and microbiology', and the general public is encouraged to 'buy shares in the test-tube baby business'.[59]

The mechanical approach to individual women's bodies is represented in the computer programmes being developed for infertility clinics. Those developed by Bailey and Associates in Oklahoma are software packages entitled 'Ovulation Induction Tracking' and 'In-Vitro Clinic +', which are 'user friendly'. But who is the user—doctor or women?

And the end result of all of this is intended to be a child. But the child has become the product of the liaison between commercial investment and medical science. Doctors discuss the '"take home" baby rate' and Harriet Blankfield's company in the US 'has five babies on the assembly line'.[60] The representation of children as products enters into the popular imagination. In Christine Nostlinger's book *Conrad. The hilarious adventures of a factory-made child*, for example, the child is delivered in a tin container.

The desire to have children or a child of a particular kind is being re-created into a need which must be satisfied: *Life* magazine refers to it as 'baby craving'.[61] Baby-making becomes just another business; as Escoffier-Lambiotte says, '[This] "medicine of desire" risks transforming medicine into a "renderer of service", with all the commercial ramifications'.[62]

Medical science and commerce are using language to create social approval for technological change which will alter reproduction on a much broader scale than 'helping the infertile' implies. Scientists themselves see this not as an important social action but as a kind of game. As American Dr Howard Jones of Norfolk says, 'it's like going to Las Vegas' trying to get 'a good egg' to meet 'a good sperm'.[63] Gena Corea has commented on the racecourse imagery involved in the competitiveness between research teams[64];

on the other hand, Hugh Niall and Geoff Tregear of the Howard Florey Institute in Melbourne discuss their work on the synthetic hormone HSG in stage comedy terms:

> 'Hugh does the sequencing (designing) and I do the synthesising: we are like a song and dance team', said Tregear. But this Rogers and Astaire of molecular biology has broken up.[65]

The scientists are also often compared to warriors and the researchers to creators of the atom bomb. Dr Alan DeCherney, Director of Reproductive Endocrinology at Yale University School of Medicine, wrote:

> How thrilling it must have been to be Chaucer writing when Gutenberg invented the printing press, or to be a physicist working on the Manhattan Project! ... an individual who is interested in fertility, who is not involved in IVF, is very similar to the West Point graduate who is educated in Military Science but never goes to war.[66]

These Boys' Own Annual pictures of scientists at work are of little comfort to women on IVF who are guinea pigs.

Perhaps, finally, we should look to language itself for an interesting perspective on the technodocs: coming from the Latin, the root of 'obstetrician', *obstet*, means 'to stand in the way'.

7. MOTHERHOOD AND INFERTILITY: MEDICAL SCIENCE CO-OPTS IDEOLOGY AND DESIRE

THE MOTHERHOOD INSTITUTION

> The mothers: collecting their children at school; sitting in rows at the parent-teacher meeting; placating weary infants in supermarket carriages; straggling home to make dinner, do laundry, and tend to children after a day at work; fighting to get decent care and livable schoolrooms for their children; waiting for child-support checks while the landlord threatens eviction; getting pregnant yet again because their one escape into pleasure and abandon is sex; forcing long needles into their delicate interior parts; wakened by a child's cry from their eternally unfinished dreams—the mothers, if we could look into their fantasies, their daydreams and imaginary experiences—we would see the embodiment of rage, of tragedy, of the overcharged energy of love, of inventive desperation, we would see the machinery of institutional violence wrenching at the experience of motherhood.[1]

When we say, 'Oh, it's a motherhood issue', we mean 'it' is unchallengeable, determined and beyond question and change. Research scientists have claimed that infertile women have the right 'to use reproductive technology programmes to attain the motherhood they so desire'. It is intimated that we are not to question that desire, nor what motherhood and mothering mean in this society.

Patriarchal science has expended considerable energy in trying to convince women that there is a 'maternal instinct'; to question motherhood is to go 'against nature'. But as Janice Raymond writes, 'It is not a woman's essence, a mystical state of being, or historically unchanging. Motherhood is whatever a given culture makes of it. It is fundamentally social, fundamentally relational...'.[2] Many women, in fact, choose not to have children.

In the past, children were born as an outcome of sexual intercourse. On many occasions this intercourse was not desired by the woman and neither were the children. It is only in the last few decades that contraception became effective enough to give women a sense of control, and in many cases the reality of control, over their procreative ability.[3] This development has a bearing on the current debates around reproductive technology, because by giving women more of a choice in childbearing, contraception allowed for the development of the desire for children in a new way. Now women can say whether they 'want' to have children. As Sichtermann has pointed out,

> In times when contraception was inadequate and unsafe, it was pure accident if pregnancy coincided with a desire to have children...People took having babies in their stride, sometimes silently pleased, sometimes just in silence, but sometimes in mute despair: they had no choice.[4]

The desire to have children has become anticipatory: it is a planned event. Women gear up mentally and emotionally in preparation for parenthood: change their lifestyle, move to a new suburb or a larger house. Ironically, because of the enlarged sense of choice which contraception brings, thwarted desire for children is harder to bear. The desire to parent becomes stronger once the decision is made, and becomes even more powerful if the choice is denied.

Motherhood is a powerful ideology in a patriarchal, pronatalist society. Leta Hollingworth wrote on 'Social Devices for Impelling Women to Bear and Rear Children'. She analysed the way in which women were coerced into having children: through the influence of public opinion; through laws for the control of women, such as sterility being legally a cause for divorce; belief about the punishment of God if families were limited; the education of women towards motherhood; the use of art to represent Madonna images of motherhood but not its negative side; the illusion that childbearing is safe and is painless; and finally what she calls 'bugaboos', such as the suggestion that delayed childbirth increases risk and that a child reared alone will become selfish and egotistic. She writes that though many democratic nations no longer practise military conscription, they 'conscript their women to bear children by legally prohibiting the publication or communication of the knowledge which would make child-bearing voluntary'. She argues that the very fact that laws have to be made against birth control, abortion, infanticide and infant desertion are proof of the 'insufficiency of maternal instinct'.[5] Hollingworth concludes by envisaging the future:

> The time is coming, and is indeed almost at hand, when all the most intelligent women of the community, who are the most desirable child-bearers, will become conscious of the methods of social control. The type of normality will be questioned; the laws will be repealed and changed; enlightenment will prevail; belief will be seen to rest upon dogmas; illusion will fade away and give place to clearness of view; the bugaboos will lose

> their power to frighten. How will 'the social guardians' induce women to bear a surplus population when all these cheap, effective methods no longer work?[6]

This clear-sighted analysis appeared in the year 1916, in the *American Journal of Sociology*. Unfortunately, Hollingworth's vision is still a little way off!

In the past, because Australia saw itself as a vulnerable 'white outpost', in danger of being overrun in an Asian area, federal governments encouraged Anglo-Celtic women to continue to produce families. Today a similar concern is apparent in debates over the immigration of people from Asian countries as opposed to European countries.

This concern about the ratio of white to non-white people is not confined to Australia: it is expressed in Western anxiety about increasing populations in so-called Third World countries and in reactions to an influx of non-white people into traditionally white living areas in places like Britain. In *The Birth Dearth* Ben Wattenberg argues that the 'free, modern, industrial world' is not replacing itself rapidly enough.[7] This is one reason for the pressure on Western women to populate, and conversely Western pressure on non-Western countries to institute and maintain population control.

Pronatalism is endemic in the white West, even in children's games where girls are taught to take on the role of mother. Assumptions are made and accepted by women and men that mothering is a natural life progression and is a necessary part of womanhood. To be a mature person is to be a parenting person, a mother. A woman makes a status passage from being a child to being an adult through her mothering. In so doing she draws upon herself various signs of social approval, both from her personal relationships (for example, her parents who expect to be grandparents) and from society in general; but this approval is not followed by a societal allocation of resources to help her do the job, nor by a socially created sense of dignity and purpose, though individual women often successfully generate these for themselves.

The assumption that child-rearing is necessary to women is reinforced and reflected in the scientific and psychological literature on development. For example, Judith Bardwick claims that there is a biological need to parent, yet after considering the evidence for and against the case, she can only write, 'I find that beneath many rational arguments one comes, finally, to a belief'. She brings out another component in the ideology of motherhood when she writes that parenting makes people mature, that it is 'moral', that it is a 'crucial existential anchor which makes people cope with real problems' and that it 'forces us to grow up'. By this analysis, people who do not parent remain immature and undeveloped. Bardwick comfortably muses that 'it is as though to some extent one of nature's fail-safe mechanisms is infertility in those who are not psychologically healthy enough to nurture'[8] (giving a scientific credibility to an offensive stereotype of the infertile person).

The prominence of motherhood for women, whether they undertake it or not, is supposedly so extensive as to affect their concept of self through the whole lifespan. Kimmel comments that 'even unmarried women often time the beginning of middle-age by the family they might have had'.[9]

In our society, women are encouraged to mother but only within the woman-man bond; both social and legal sanctions have been imposed on women who have children outside marriage. Thus we have the 'motherhood continuum of heterosexual intercourse, pregnancy, and childraising as compulsory for women'.[10] This is not a thing of the past. Legislation passed to date concerning reproductive technology, for example in England and Australia, makes these technologies available only to women in a 'stable heterosexual relationship'. In Victorian legislation, single and lesbian women are excluded, and this is true in many countries with respect to the simple procedures of artificial insemination. This reflects men's anxiety that women may take childbearing out of the heterosexual/family structure; a structure which has institutionalised women's economic dependence and service duties towards men (physically, sexually and emotionally).

SHAPING WOMEN AND THEIR EXPERIENCES OF MOTHERHOOD AND SELF

Part of the definition of motherhood in a patriarchal society is one of self-denying and self-sacrificing love. In Chapter 4 'surrogates' repeatedly indicated their willingness to sacrifice self for another. Not only the definition of woman, but the definition of mother takes on these characteristics of self-denial and martyrdom. Women are supposed to experience life in the public sphere vicariously through their husbands, and to get their sense of achievement vicariously through their children: 'our stamp upon the world has been, traditionally, our stamp upon our children'.[11] The 'selflessness' of women has led to a devastating self-debasement and the martyrdom of many mothers, which children gradually learn to resent.

Davies and Welch discuss how the 'tyranny of happiness' became established in the ideology of motherhood after the 1950s. The intensity of the mother–child bond was encouraged within an increasingly limited nuclear family setting where the 'ethic of care' slid into the 'ethic of self-sacrifice'. As one mother said:

> I keep feeling that I'm not contributing outside the household and it really gets to me. Well, I just feel as

> though I am just marking time, I am not doing anything that is useful to anybody apart from maintaining the house and Mark [the child]... I just dropped out of the whole world.

Davies and Welch place the responsibility for the negative experience of motherhood firmly within the institutional and ideological structures that control it:

> Thus it is not the mothering of small children or motherhood *per se* that makes for such ambivalence on the part of those involved. It is doing it under certain conditions (in the isolation of a nuclear family) and with a particular set of beliefs about womanhood combined with beliefs about motherhood. There are certain consequences accruing from these beliefs and conditions—the over-riding one being a potential loss of self.[12]

Many women experience depression when they face an unexpected decrease in power simply because of child-bearing.[13] Regardless of the ideological reification of motherhood, once women enter into its boundaries there is little power, as it is experienced in the public sphere, to be exercised. Men do not enter into the rearing of children because

> as an unpaid occupation outside the world of public power, [parenting] entails lower status, less power, and less control of resources than paid work. Women's mothering reinforces and perpetuates women's relative powerlessness.[14]

Their work socialising the next generation is not seen as worthy of comment or of payment.

Although women are deemed to be instinctively mothers, men also create an aura of female incompetence around motherhood; women carry the responsibility for the work of child-rearing, while authority about how it should be done is in the hands of men, leading to the 'deskilling' of mothers. In Australia, as in other countries, concern about infant mortality rates and population size at the turn of the century gave medical practitioners and scientists a justification for intervening in the mothering process to ensure 'more efficient' mothering.

Whatever their decisions about their lives women cannot escape having to make decisions about, or relating in some way to, motherhood: motherhood is the 'great mesh in which all human relations are entangled'.[15] Hence, 'the idea of *choice*... is almost beyond our grasp. Our thoughts and actions are shaped by the most deeply ingrained notions of what we "ought" to do; knowing what we want is not as simple as it may seem'.[16]

But women do resist both motherhood itself and the negative experience which patriarchy has defined as appropriate. Adrienne Rich has drawn a distinction between the institution of motherhood as men have defined it and as described above, and the '*potential relationship* of any woman to her powers of reproduction and to children'.[17] Sara Ruddick articulates the difficulty of mothering for women in patriarchy. She writes:

> Almost everywhere, the practices of mothering take place in societies in which women of all classes are less powerful than men of their class to determine the conditions under which their children grow. Throughout history, most women have mothered in conditions of military and social violence and often of extreme poverty. They have been governed by men, and increasingly by managers and experts of both sexes, whose policies mothers neither shape nor control.[18]

In their role of socialising children mothers are expected to encourage the children to be obedient to the dominant patriarchal values. 'This may mean training her daughters for powerlessness, her sons for war, and both for crippling work in dehumanising factories, businesses and professions'.[19]

On the other hand, motherhood has 'compensated for a great deal of the oppression women experience inside and outside their homes'.[20] Women often seek in mothering an intimacy of experience which men are unable to give. Irena Klepfisz expresses this:

> When depressed about the fragility and transience of friendships or the inconsistencies of lovers, it was the myth of a child, a blood relation and what it would bring me, which seemed to me the only real guarantee against loneliness and isolation, the only way of maintaining a connection to the rest of society.[21]

Of course in many instances this ideal is not fulfilled for the women concerned: their children may be uncaring and disconnected. But for many that reciprocal love and sense of intimacy with another human being, that sense of continuity in relationship, is a real impetus towards having children. Motherhood is also seen by women as giving them an experience of power and control in a world which does not offer this experience to women in most spheres. And there is the sense of sharing with other mothers. Barbara Wishart, an Australian lesbian mother, writes that

> The experience of motherhood has given me a deep bond with other mothers I know, and a sense of continuity not only with the women in my own family, but also with a continuous line of women from antiquity to the present day who have borne children.[22]

There is the physical experience of mothering; not only giving birth, though pregnancy, birth and breast feeding are, of course, unique intimate physical relationships with another human being, but the physical relationship in the rearing of a child, in the bathing and daily caring routines. Because women have been made solely responsible for child-rearing, for the most part this physical relationship with children remains a female experience.

As well as resisting the patriarchal negativism of mothering, women have resisted motherhood itself historically by choosing not to have children. Often they are seen as unlikeable, selfish and uncaring child-haters. In one study of community attitudes in the US researchers asked their respondents to judge the personality and character of both child-free couples and couples with children. People perceived the sterilised child-free wife as 'less sensitive and loving, less typical an American woman, more likely to be active in women's liberation, and less happy, less well adjusted, less likely to get along with her parents, and less likely to be happy and satisfied at age 65' than an identically described mother of two.[23]

Generally the advantages which women see in remaining child-free are: they will not experience the career and job disadvantage of time out of the workforce; they can continue a freer lifestyle which involves travel and job mobility; and they will not risk interference with and erosion of the intimacy of their marriage relationship. They feel that a family life denies them equality and would impose upon them the 'appropriate' sex-typed stereotypes. They express a strong desire for self-development. One seventy-three-year-old child-free woman wrote in 1982:

> If you want to know what it is like to grow older without children I will tell you, it is marvellous. My neighbour, older than I and a friend younger than I, all without children, time and time again say to one another, 'thank goodness I never had children'. Never once has any of us ever regretted it, and many other times we have rejoiced over it... we were the smart ones.[24]

For some women, 'choice' within male-defined motherhood is no choice, so they exercise their own will and resist the role of mother. For them, this resistance becomes 'the ultimate liberation'.[25]

This decision is not an easy one to make as women come under pressure from parents to present grandchildren and to be part of the generational process. Friends of their own generation tend to begin having families and drop out of social contact. They experience periods of regret and re-assessment which are often triggered by Christmas or a birthday. Moreover, there are many social and institutional sanctions which constantly remind them that they are odd and out of step with the rest of society. Child-free women are constantly resented, slighted and socially isolated from families with children on the assumption that they dislike children and in some cases as a form of punishment for their choice.

WOMEN'S EXPERIENCE OF INFERTILITY IN PATRIARCHY

But what of the women who, because of fertility problems which they or their partners have, remain involuntarily childless? Infertility has been a taboo subject for a long time and women have taken the blame in childless relationships. Men are never assumed to be 'the problem'. Focusing on infertility through reproductive technology has not shifted these negative attitudes, but rather highlighted the woman-blaming aspects of it. Women are stigmatised as 'desperate' and as 'willing to do anything' if they are infertile. (Rarely do we hear of those infertile women who have adjusted to their situation and moved on in life to the next goal.) These women want to mother because of the joys they expect the experience to bring, as outlined above. But it is also hardly surprising that women are torn and driven by infertility when that experience takes place within a pronatalist patriarchal society.

Women are usually tested first in infertility regimes, even though the tests may be more painful and onerous for them than for men. Women are blamed for infertility as if it were a punishment. They are accused of having sexually transmitted diseases, of having been promiscuous, or having had too many abortions. In a revealing comment the Director of the Sterility Clinic at the Women's Hospital in Crown Street, Sydney, was quoted as saying,

> In my experience—and I became interested in this subject 30 years ago—a very large percentage of infertility problems in women are self-inflicted. There are, of course, many cases that are just bad luck.[26]

Sometimes the woman is said to have 'hostile mucus', or an 'allergic reaction' to sperm. Against this, Hull et al. suggest in the *Lancet* that 'defective sperm function is a frequent hidden cause of infertility':

> The Edinburgh study comparing sperm/mucus penetration in vitro and hamster egg penetration confirms that the defect resides in the sperm, not in the mucus or egg. The usual terms 'cervical infertility' and 'mucus hostility' are therefore inappropriate.[27]

The facts are that in a third of infertile couples the problem is traceable to the woman, a further third are traceable to the man and in the remaining third the cause is unknown.[28]

Many women have infertility problems because of contraceptive devices used in the past and many are infertile because of iatrogenic or doctor-induced problems. Dr William Keye warned gynaecologists that 'we may cause more infertility than we care to believe' based on the 36 per cent rate of doctor-induced problems in one hospital which he described as common. In one study of 65 women with pelvic disease at a US infertility clinic, 38.5 per cent had undergone previous obstetric and gynaecological procedures that might have contributed to their fertility problem.[29] In another analysis of 206 infertile women, 75 per cent were found to have had previous pelvic surgery which could account for their infertility. Dr John Musich, Chairman of the Department of Obstetrics and Gynaecology at Wayne State University, warned medicos that any operations near the pelvis could threaten fertility.[30]

Warnings appear again and again in the pages of *Ob. Gyn. News.* Apart from post-operative infection which can occur due to poor treatment after abortion or pelvic operations, women can also suffer from adhesions and scarring due to poor operative technique. One of the major problems for women is a tubal problem, and fallopian tubes may be blocked by infection from using IUDs, scarring, or of course sterilisation. Pelvic inflammatory disease is also a major threat to women's fertility. The risk of contracting PID is four to nine times higher in women with an IUD than in those without.[31]

Other causes of infertility in women may be related to herbicides and pesticides. One study in Austria and Germany found evidence of fungicide, insecticides and PCB in the eggs and follicular fluid of women undergoing IVF. More and more environmental toxins are becoming named as a source of infertility in both women and men.[32]

Blaming women for infertility adds to the burden which pronatalism and the motherhood mandate have already imposed on their sense of self. Something over which they felt they had control they did not. The search for a remedy through reproductive technology leads them to a further loss of self-esteem and added pain, as I showed in Chapter 1. Infertility can batter the self-definition of a woman. One woman felt 'emotionally distraught, worthless, extremely upset, and angry. It was bitter disappointment, social rejection—a feeling of being incomplete'.[33] Another wrote, 'It affected my self-esteem, it made me feel depressed for at least 12 months, it affected our relationship, it affected my sexuality. I felt powerless'.[34]

Infertile women often feel overwhelmed with guilt. This was true for thirty of the forty women Renate Klein talked to. One woman felt guilty 'because I was involuntarily withholding something that had become very important to him. I also felt guilt about an abortion at sixteen'. Since many people marry in order to create a family, they feel confused about what the relationship now means. One woman said, 'I was certainly looking for somebody who would be a father as well as a husband. And he was certainly looking for a mother of his child as well'.[35]

Following the medical profession's lead in defining their bodies as defective and worthless if they cannot reproduce, many women take on a negative self-image and body image. One said, 'I felt my body was cheating me. It had let me down'. Another said:

> I didn't like my body. It [infertility] makes you very contemptuous. Even though I don't think breasts are only for breast feeding... when you're thinking... any month, when you are looking forward to breast feeding in nine or ten months, you don't like your breasts either. It really does have an effect on your body image.

Infertile women often describe themselves as 'hollow', 'empty', 'barren' or 'wasted and arid'. But there is also a debate about the use of the word 'infertile'. Anne Aitken rejects the word. She says,

> Although I have a fertility problem, I am not an infertile woman. I hate the word infertile. It is used to describe a paddock in the country. It's infertile, it won't produce anything. I am a productive person in a lot of ways.

> I don't have to have a child to prove I'm as good as other women.[36]

In a pronatalist society largely structured around the nuclear family, childless women feel isolated and lonely. Often people conspire not to talk about pregnancies of friends or families, thus denying the infertile woman the adult status of dealing with her own responses to these situations. Pregnant friends often stop calling in order not to inflict hurt, unaware that it is more hurtful to imply a lack of interest or an overinterest on the part of an infertile friend than to bring the discussion of the issue into the open. Infertile women often feel they have failed physically and socially.

POWER AND RESISTANCE: HOW WOMEN SHAPE THE EXPERIENCES OF INFERTILITY AND MOTHERHOOD

Regaining control of the infertility experience is as difficult for women as shaping motherhood. The power of desire denied is one of the most difficult of human passions. To refuse medical techniques which seem to offer a quick fix takes enormous courage and faith in self.

Infertile women and many feminists have begun by looking at the real causes of infertility in an effort to displace the woman-blaming of our society. They find that there is little emphasis placed on preventing infertility and little on looking at holistic methods of dealing with women's fertility problems. For example, findings which indicate that excessive exercise or stress of any kind influences women's ovulation and menstruation as well as the production of sperm could lead to behavioural changes which might solve a fertility problem.[37]

Women are also looking at the connection between mind and body, refusing to accept science's mind/body split. It is possible that some women do not conceive because they are relaying various messages, emotionally and mentally, to the body, in order to block ovulation. I talked to a woman who already had a child but was supposedly not ovulating; her doctor had put her on clomiphene citrate. It emerged that she had had a stillbirth nine months previously and had had no counselling or discussions with anyone about it. It became obvious that the woman was suffering from severe grief and anxiety that, should she conceive again, the child would die. After four sessions of therapy she became pregnant naturally.

Paul Entwistle, a researcher in scientific aspects of infertility at Liverpool University and a counsellor and hypnotherapist, asserts that of the 200 patients he has seen that have unsuccessfully tried conventional fertility treatments, 65 per cent conceived after hypnotherapy. He believes that many women and many men think they want a baby but subconsciously do not.

> I have been seeing a couple who have tried in vitro fertilisation five times. You would think they must be 100 per cent committed to a pregnancy to go through all that. But as we talked, it gradually became obvious that wasn't the case.

Entwistle often meets women who have lost a baby through abortion, miscarriage or stillbirth and have not finished their grieving process. He also comes across patients who experience guilt which can block the fertility process. He comments that 'if a woman has subconsciously chosen to be infertile while trying for a baby, she may switch off her fertility in some ways'.[38]

These comments do not mean that infertility is 'all in the mind', but for many women there is no legitimate way to avoid mothering apart from being infertile. It may be that a woman is satisfied with her life and does not want to move into motherhood, yet the social pressure of family, friends and husband make it difficult to resist: the mind then finds a way of taking care of the problem at another level.

The need for counselling and support is evident. Though the support groups which are attached to reproductive technology programmes in Australia are useful to some people, others see them as merely keeping up the spirits of 'failed patients' and keeping them on the 'lookout for new technologies that, perhaps, might work'.[39]

Alison Solomon (herself infertile) describes infertility crisis counselling in Israel which could be a more useful model to follow.[40] Geraldine Stevens, an infertile woman and founder of such a group in Australia, found that not all women with a fertility problem want children, but want to come to grips with the fact that they do have a fertility problem. For many women, recovering their health or fertility is more important than the desire for a child, and the loss of control marked by a fertility problem is a more important issue for many women than the inability to have their own child. She found that many women were being pushed onto IVF against their wishes. Stevens became involved herself in a shared parenting arrangement and argues that many women would be happy with access to social parenting. What is needed is a way of breaking the stranglehold of the nuclear family so that those who are interested in parenting may join with parents in that.

Ultimately people need to resolve major disappointments, frustrations and painful experiences in life. Women are setting limits on what they are prepared to do to try to overcome their infertility. Many women refuse to enter into invasive technological programmes; others set limits as to how long they are prepared to undergo these procedures. Toni Chapman set a time limit of two and a half years for trying to conceive a child. In the end she felt that taking her temperature every morning as the first act of the day only served to remind her of her failure to conceive. On her thirtieth birthday she had a ceremonial smashing of her thermometer. That milestone brought a sense of relief:

> I could start to lead my life again, work hard, go on holidays, decide about our house. I want to live a life that is most productive socially and most satisfying personally. That goal is certainly not filled by seeking vainly one of the ways I can live my life—as a mother. Other roles are more easily attained in my case.[41]

Among many letters written to the National Association for the Childless in England was one from a man of eighty-eight:

> Nobody has ever called me father or grandfather. I am now alone with the memories that other people pass on to their children. I am not afraid. I am a father you see. Not to a person, but to those things I caused to be, the furniture I made, the people who relied on me. I wish you well with your Association, but never make the mistake of believing the childless are not parents. All carry that love—there are many paths to follow.

In her epilogue to *Coping with Childlessness,* Diane Houghton, a childless woman married for twenty years, said she found it hard to 'invest with great emotion' the period when she was so distressed by her grief at childlessness, so happy and satisfied has her life turned out to be. She found that to be fully occupied in demanding and satisfying work helped to salve the disappointment of infertility. She pointed out that having children would not necessarily ameliorate the problems of age. Most importantly she points out that 'in some ways, perhaps, the choice is made easier in that these tempting miracle solutions [reproductive technology] were not dangled before me'.[42]

THE FUTURE OF MOTHERHOOD

As Adrienne Rich has written: 'Mothering and nonmothering have been such charged concepts for us, precisely because *whichever we did has been turned against us*'.[43] Yet even 'with all the conflicts and contradictions, women have succeeded at mothering'.[44] Adrienne Rich maintains hope for what motherhood may be, redefined by women, because of

> ...all that we have managed to salvage, of ourselves, for our children, even within the destructiveness of the institution: the tenderness, the passion, the trust in our instincts, the evocation of a courage we did not know we owned, the detailed apprehension of another human existence, the full realization of the cost and precariousness of life.[45]

She argues for the destruction of the institution of motherhood as it is currently defined.

> To destroy the institution is not to abolish motherhood. It is to release the creation and sustenance of life into the same realm of decision, struggle, surprise, imagination, and conscious intelligence, as any other difficult, but freely chosen work.[46]

Janice Raymond also emphasises that mothering is only one of a range of women's skills, but that

> unless we question motherhood as an institution, unless we question its compulsory nature and its overriding centrality in women's lives, unless we critique the notion that women's main fulfillment is through mothering and nurturing, unless we realise that for many women motherhood is not a choice, but something that has been imposed within a social and political order of hetero-relations (the worldview that women exist for men and only in relation to them) we end up valorizing motherhood

> without criticizing the foundations on which it has been built. That is why I would not stress women's collective power in procreation.

Motherhood itself is not a social power base. Men desire to control it, as if it were powerful, and women resist this control. Rightly, women judge that if men so desire it, it must give them some power in relations between the sexes. But control of this area alone does not lead to empowerment. Raymond argues that 'women will not have collective power in procreation unless women have collective power in other areas of life'.[47]

FATHER-RIGHT: THE MALE RESPONSE

When women challenge the patriarchal definitions of mothering and infertility, male control slips; but through a blend of reproductive technology and legal means, men as a group and as individuals are reasserting 'rights' over children and women. Definitions of 'mother' and 'father' are a crucial part of this and it is motherhood which is thrown into confusion.

Mothering has always been experienced by women in terms of relationship. To deny the birth mother's real experience of relationship with her developing fetus and resulting child is wrong. For women, the relationship is complex—she is not just a capsule carrying a developing seed; the fetus that is growing is intimately linked with her body. Mothering can also be the rearing of a child, and a mother who is rearing a child not genetically related to her has also formed a *relationship* with the child. But the genetic donor has not necessarily done this.

For men, the concept of fathering has been concerned primarily with the ownership of children. The new reproductive technologies reinforce this, as stress is constantly placed on who owns the embryos created through IVF. This point is further emphasised in the attitudes of couples using artificial insemination by donor and IVF. Lasker and Borg found that of those filling out their questionnaires,

> men usually appear to be the driving force behind the preference for a biological child. Many women told us they would be happy to adopt, but their husbands wanted a genetic connection. The men agreed... Genes are the biggest contribution men make to the creation of a child. They cannot carry, birth, or nurse a baby. In addition, they are rarely the major care-giver. Women can 'mother' in many ways. Many men... focus on the biological connection.[48]

As one woman said in explaining her husband's reluctance to adopt a child, 'He says he just couldn't accept an adopted child as his own'.[49]

Through the new technologies, as Barbara Katz Rothman has pointed out, women are being made, in a sense, into fathers. Discussing egg donation she writes: 'But looking at it another way, the donor is not a mother at all. She is a father: she contributes half of the genetic material, her "seed".[50]

In so-called surrogacy, it is the birth mother's relationship to the child which is the basis of her claim to her or him. This relationship is 'based on her contribution to the child'. In contrast, as Janice Raymond argues, the sperm donor who battles for ownership of a child in a surrogacy case, claiming to be a 'father' has not made a contribution to the fetus becoming a child equal to the birth mother's. 'The father does not assume the risks of conception, pregnancy and birth, nor does he do the work of carrying the fetus for nine months'. Yet in the surrogacy debate, the giving of sperm has been made equal to the contribution of the egg, gestation and birthing.[51]

Father-right gives rights and privileges to a man over children who come from his sperm but for whom he often shows minimal responsibility. As women increasingly become economically independent and increasingly produce children outside the heterosexual marriage situation, so legal changes are made to ensure that the man from whom the sperm comes has rights over those children.

Outlining legal changes foreshadowed in Britain, Sutton and Friedman conclude that 'what has resulted is a minimal change in caring and a significant move by men to increase their rights and hence, control'. They write that women in the 150 refuges for battered women in England will attest that 'when a man has access to a child, he is able to use the child to further his own interests and to control that child's mother'.[52] Increased father-right, instead of increasing paternal responsibility for children, legally enforces the concept of women and children as belonging to men. Recent legislation in many other countries including New Zealand, Switzerland, France, the former West Germany and many Australian states has extended the rights of fatherhood to men whose children are born outside marriage.[53]

Internationally, most men fail to pay for the maintenance and support of their children after a divorce. The prevalent attitude is that a man need only be responsible while he has overt control over them and over the woman, but once the woman claims independence from the man, he often denies his obligation to the children or he uses his payments to try to regain control.

In Australia in 1983 it was suggested that men should be forced to pay maintenance for their children through tighter court procedures. A number of men's groups rose up in response to this suggestion. Glenn Martin, a Justice of the Peace, wrote to the *National Times:*

> I think mothers have to be quite clear about what they

> are expecting... If they choose to leave a man then they have to become responsible for their own lives and for those of their children. If they want maintenance they should realise that it is humanly impossible for any such money to be free of other links with the man.
>
> If the man leaves, it's no different. If you want the man to be responsible, you have got to see that in terms of personal involvement with the children, and not just as maintenance. And if the man doesn't want to be involved you have to consider that maybe you're better off anyway, even without his money.[54]

Many women have in fact decided that they are better off without this connection and struggle to support their children without accepting money which necessitates contact with the father.

In 1986, the Australian federal government released proposals on its intention to collect maintenance at the source; that is, directly from the supporting parent through his/her pay cheque. Statistics indicated that only one in ten single mothers receive maintenance. Again men were quick to respond. Patrick Heffernan, from Parents Without Rights, a primarily male organisation, said that fathers should pay only if they received the reward of services of a wife and access to their children. The men he represents are mainly those who 'have been denied access to their children by the courts, or by wives on the run from them'. He worried that 85 per cent of 'these women' have a boyfriend with a car who has 'taken on the pleasure of a relationship, and has stepped in to fill the former husband's role'. This man, he argues, should 'take on the responsibility for that woman and her [*sic*] children'.[55]

Mother-right, in contrast, is not enshrined within the law. So the 'illegitimate' child, in English and Australian common law, was defined as a child of no one. It was paternity which gave the child status, not maternity. In her extensive eight-year analysis of custody battles in sixty-five countries, Phyllis Chesler found that 'maternal right' has never been legitimised. She documents the brutality of these legal battles and shows that mothers are rarely judged 'good enough' to keep their children in cases where custody arrangements come into question. The more traditional a woman has been—a 'good' mother in patriarchal terms—the weaker her grounds for custody because of her financial dependence.[56] The intention of the law is to reinforce father-right.

Carol Smart traces the development of the laws relating to paternity in England. She points out that before the Children Act of 1975, fathers were quick to disown illegitimate children because of the costs that would result in being required to contribute financially to their care. This began to change when it was realised that unmarried mothers were on the increase; women having children outside the control of men. The Law Commission's working paper on illegitimacy in 1979 was actually a document arguing against the wrongs seen to be done to unmarried fathers. Smart writes:

> The Commission lists all the discriminations 'suffered' by the unmarried father and concludes that the best method of eradicating these wrongs and eliminating the problem of illegitimacy, was to give all biological fathers automatic paternal rights on a par with the mother of an illegitimate child. Under this proposal the unmarried mother would have to go to the court if she wanted sole custody or did not wish the father to exercise his rights. These rights include not only actual custody, but the right to decide whether the child should have medical treatment, which school the child should go to, where the child should live and what the child's

name should be.

The Commission later abandoned these proposals because of the adverse reactions they received, but in its later recommendations of 1982 it did not 'rescind the proposal that all fathers should have the right to be named'. AID donors, however, were excluded because they were not the men who would accept the financial obligation of paternity.

Considering the laws on divorce, Smart points out that the presumption that courts favour mothers now when dealing with custody of children is incorrect and that they usually only give legal recognition to those arrangements decided by the parents themselves. New moves have put pressure on the courts to award parental rights jointly to both parents. Under this arrangement the responsibility for everyday care would still be with the mother, but the father would have control over decisions about schooling and so on: authority remains with the father. Smart comments:

> This development (see the Booth Committee Report, 1985) is, like the developments on illegitimacy, linked to a disquiet about the power of mothers if they have sole custody. It is feared that the bitterness of the mother may deny a child the right to know and see its father.

She points out that when the law starts discussing the 'best interests of the child', it is usually concerning itself with the rights of fathers.

In a further interesting example of the emphasis on paternal rights, she notes that the Warnock Committee Report on human fertilisation and embryology (1985) recommended that the government should actively discourage a woman from using the frozen semen of her dead husband for insemination and that a frozen embryo should not be implanted in the wife if the husband is dead. But there are no recommendations against using

> these same methods where the husband is alive but where the biological mother is dead. Should a widower elect to implant the egg or embryo of his dead wife into an infertile second wife, the child born as a consequence will not be disinherited or ignored for the purposes of succession.[57]

Looking at the increased role of fathers in child care, there is a similar delineation between mothers taking responsibility for children and fathers wielding authority. 'They do not come into child rearing as workers, they come in as managers whose decision-making power is derived from the structures of sexual inequality'. Men play with children rather than work at the more mundane jobs.[58]

As I indicated in Chapter 4, father-right is most clear in battles over custody between so-called surrogates (birth mothers) and their sperm donors (deemed to be 'fathers'). Judge Sorkow in the Whitehead case ruled that Stern was not buying the child because '*he cannot purchase what is already his*'. But, as Raymond points out, '*she* [Whitehead] cannot change her mind about what is already hers because, in effect, it is his and not hers. Sperm plus money doth a father make.' Sorkow wrote 'To this day she [Whitehead] still appears to reject any role Mr Stern played in the conception. She chooses to forget that *but for him there would be no child*'.[59] Here the sperm donor is elevated to the role of father, while the biological and birth mother becomes a bit-part actor in the drama.

Increasingly men are attempting to legitimate their authority over women and children through claims to biological fatherhood. This concept of male ownership extends more and more now to fetal life as well. In England a university student requested an injunction to stop his pregnant former girlfriend from having an abortion, on the grounds that it would amount to child destruction under the Infant Life (Preservation) Act of 1929. The case turned on the issue of whether the fetus could be defined as a child; that is, was it capable of being born alive; it did not revolve around the rights of the woman. The man had no intention of rearing the child. His intention merely was to ensure that 'his child' was born. He wanted to make the woman carry the child to term and have it adopted.[60]

Men continue to battle for control over women, children and the processes of procreation while women with children continue to resist both male control and the current unfulfilling definitions of motherhood. For the infertile woman, turning her inability to bear children into a positive experience is even more difficult, and it becomes more painful as reproductive technology gives its false promise of happiness if she will only cling to motherhood as meaning in life and 'try everything'.

The relationship between medical science and commerce outlined in preceding chapters has shown that science cannot afford to cure infertility. Research emphasises the high-tech response and neglects prevention. Scientists claim that they do all this because 'women want it'. But what is desire created in the context of mandatory motherhood? And what is choice?

8. RIGHTS, RESPONSIBILITIES AND RESISTANCE

DESIRE BECOMES 'RIGHTS'

In 1988, Chet Fleming created debate in the *British Medical Journal* with his book on keeping a severed head 'alive'. Fleming took out a 'prophetic patent' in the US in order to stop such an idea being followed through without adequate discussion. He cited experiments in which transplanted monkey heads had been kept 'alive' for thirty-six hours:

> I have been contacted by half a dozen people who want to know how soon the operation will be available and how much it will cost. Some are dying; others are paralysed. Most said that if the mind remains clear and the head can still think, remember, see, read, hear, and talk and if the operation leads to numbness rather than pain below the neck they would want it.[1]

This is not cited here to foretell of a world of transplanted body parts, though that is no longer unimaginable. The question which arises here is that if desire (want) is generated by technological possibility or reality, is that sufficient to justify pursuit of that technique by science? I think not.

Busy with the 'realities' of work, relationships and the daily grind, we often unquestioningly accept what it is we are told we want, and leave unchallenged many assumptions about the ways we should behave and feel. Yet because of the social origins of many of these wants and desires, they can be challenged and changed; the coercive impact of ideologies such as patriarchy and capitalism can be resisted. Many women's voices in this book have already told that story.

This is not to say that desire should always be denied because it is socially determined. But it does mean that we can question technodocs, and indeed the users of technology who claim a 'right' to use it on behalf of women, as if it is in 'the nature of things', as if the right is owed to them by society.[2] Just wanting something is no grounds for receiving it. Yet the fulfilment of desire is more and more couched in the language of rights—a word which implies a *moral* justification.

The notion of individual rights comes from a liberal stream of philosophical thought, currently particularly prominent in the US, which has been part of libertarian philosophy, although in Europe and Australia the term contractarianism is more applicable (in these places 'libertarian' refers to the anarchist wing of the socialist movement).[3] The 'individual' discussed in these philosophies is paramount and is sexless. This in itself should be a red flag of warning to feminists, who understand particularly well that there are *male* individuals and *female* individuals. Moreover, these 'rights' exist within a patriarchal value system. They include the right to 'free trade': the right to exercise power over others; the right to privacy (often defined as raping or beating your wife); the right to use and create pornography; the right of women to work as prostitutes but not as company managers, and finally the right to use force to get what you want ('might is right'). Patriarchal values rarely address the *responsibilities* of men, either to each other or to society as a whole, or to women.

A conceptualisation of rights underpinned by feminist

values would stress very different things, like the right to clean air, clean food and water, to adequate housing, health and education; to caring relationships; to draw on communal resources when necessary; to human dignity and bodily integrity; to be free of coercion in childbearing; and to freedom from assault, fear and terror. As Harrison writes:

> ... a society that incorporates a perdurable structure of coercion, even violence, against women as morally appropriate to its functioning but claims that it upholds the sanctity of or respect for human life is deluded.[4]

The concept of individual rights has been used by feminists in order to gain some measure of equality; in societies where the individual has become deified, the rhetoric of rights was a useful tool in feminist demands for equality. Unfortunately, it has often led to battles around equal rights but not equality of outcome.

It is understandable that in a society where so much has been denied to individual women, we would turn towards individualism in a desire to find autonomy and integrity. But we need to be wary, for individualism, closely tied to ownership, is 'the fulcrum on which modern patriarchy turns'.[5] Feminists prefer to stress sharing and collectivity.

Though some advances have been made within the strictures of a libertarian individualism, women are still far from experiencing autonomy and integrity. In her analysis of the law in the US, Catharine MacKinnon points out that though there has been legislation guaranteeing pay equality, women are still the greatest number of the poor, and pay is far from being sex-equal. Though feminists have been part of the move for making divorce easier, more women are losing custody of their children. Though rape is constantly increasing, convictions for rape are not. Though some legal advances are being made against sexual harassment and domestic violence, MacKinnon argues that the 'string of defeats and declines' which feminism comes up against makes us realise that liberal thinking and liberal law go only part way towards the struggle for women's equality: 'the abstract equality of liberalism permits most women little more than does the substantive inequality of conservatism'.[6]

If society is viewed as merely a collection of individuals, all of whom have their 'rights', there is no concept of the public good or interdependent relationships with other people. Women have quite rightly been wary of 'interdependence' because it has always been defined by patriarchy as women's economic and man's emotional dependence. When people in our society are asked to put their own individual desire aside for the public good, it is women who are usually to put *their* needs to one side while the well-being of men has been defined as the 'public good'.

Trying to find a way round these dilemmas in her work on abortion, Beverley Wildung Harrison argues that ' "rights" in a moral sense, then, are shares in the basic conditions of human well-being and, therefore, *reciprocal accountabilities* that are binding for all persons' (my emphasis).[7] The concept of rights must be tempered with this accountability and responsibility to the social group. Though this has always been defined unjustly in such a way as to make women alone ultimately responsible for the well-being of the social group while denying themselves, we must develop a theory and a practice based on both individual integrity and social accountability, particularly to women but also to society.

There are crucial differences between arguments for the right to reproductive freedom with respect to abortion/ contraception, and the so-called right to use reproductive technology couched in the same rhetoric. Women must have the right *not* to reproduce and mother because the alternative would mean that they are *compelled* to do so. Coerced motherhood is an assault on woman and child. Access to safe contraception and abortion, as yet not achieved by all women in *any* country, is essential to a woman's autonomy. She must have the right to reproduce free from enforced sterilisation or forced abortion. On the other hand, there can be no concomitant right to have a child: the right to live without bodily coercion is not the same as the 'right' to draw on community funds or resources as if one were *owed* a child/product. Likewise a man does not have the 'right' to use a woman as a so-called surrogate because he has a 'right' to the child/product. As Rosalind Petchesky has noted, 'there will remain a *level of individual desire that can never be totally reconciled with social need*'.[8]

Women often mistake individualism for autonomy and believe that using the terminology of rights will achieve this. But it is ultimately a self-only approach, a solipsistic and isolated picture of society. As Susan Sherwin puts it:

> As I understand feminism, it is committed to developing a spirit of co-operation, fostering healthy human interaction, and ensuring a sense of mutual responsibility among persons. The autonomy feminism embraces is a freedom from dominance, a liberation from aggression, and not mere isolation and separation.[9]

THE NATURE OF CHOICE

Within a rights-based approach to reproductive technologies, technodocs and users alike argue that women should be able to make a 'free' choice to use a technology. They claim that opponents of the technology want to deny women choice and are treating women as if they are stupid and 'brainwashed' by social custom.[10]

In analysing the constraints on women's so-called choices,

I am not saying that women are weak and manipulated; I am not denying women integrity and agency in our society. Rather I am recognising the way power works and the masculine values which determine the so-called free choices available. The arguments that 'I have the right to' and 'I am capable of making choices' are very seductive in our current ideological framework. Yet those statements are made as if we live in some kind of pure environment where there are no power dynamics and no hierarchies, and they are based in a false assumption of freedom. Moreover, there is a danger that the claim to rights and free choice can be, as Petchesky has said, perverted into a bourgeois individualism, justifying selfishness[11]; women may become complacent about their own sense of individual power, neglecting their obligations to women as a social group and to the social change we need to ensure better welfare for women and men.

We need to move away from simplistic claims to personal autonomy and choice to consider the nature of choice itself. It is usually thought of as a decision freely made between positive alternatives. The illusion of 'free' choice gives us a sense of personal control over our lives but ignores hierarchies in the society in which we live. The term is used in interesting colloquial ways: as in 'Hobson's Choice'—taking the first horse in the stable or none at all, which is what having children used to be like, or in 'Sophie's Choice'—choosing between equally unpleasant or negative alternatives, which is what amniocentesis revealing an 'abnormal' fetus gives women now, the 'choice' between having a disabled child with special needs, or aborting. As Robin Morgan wrote:

> We are told that freedom is synonymous with choice; yet what *is* choice to the shopper in the supermarket who can have her pick of twenty different breakfast

> cereals (all made by the same company) or to the student who can train for any career but (depending on the shape or shade of one's skin) have access to few? What is choice to the Hindu widow who faced either death on her husband's funeral pyre or a life of ostracism and slow starvation? What is choice to the voter in a one-party election—or in a two-party system where both parties articulate virtually the same politics, but with ingeniously different rhetoric? Who defines the choices among which we choose?[12]

In reproductive technology the 'choice' presented to infertile women is either to live the life of thc infertile with all the social stigma and negativity which is currently attached to that, or to undergo abusive, violent and dangerous procedures in the attempt to have a child. This is not choice as feminists would construct it.

Women do have agency—I do not deny their decision-making powers—but their decisions are made within a social context, constrained and shaped by the forces of economics, social ideology, personal psychology, and established power structures. These decisions are hedged around by structured constraints depending on a woman's race, class, age, marital status, sexuality, religion, culture and able-bodiedness, and the constraints are greater for women than for men. We do not live in a world with no power imbalances. We live in a world structured around hierarchies with some people deliberately given more advantages than others.

There is no equality in the alternatives offered to people as 'choices' and no equality between those who are 'choosing'. The choices of some individuals are firmly based upon the lack of choice of others. Often women who are comfortably situated in their own lives forget the reality of power differences, become blinded to the insidious nature of oppression, feeling themselves safe and unfettered. Many experience a considerable measure of choice and control in their own lives and mistake it for the real liberation of all women. As Bell Hooks warns:

> Many women in this society do have choices (as inadequate as they are) therefore exploitation and discrimination are words that more accurately describe the lot of women collectively in the United States... they may know they are discriminated against on the basis of sex, but they do not equate this with oppression... the absence of extreme restrictions lead many women to ignore the areas in which they are exploited or discriminated against; it may even lead them to imagine that no women are oppressed.[13]

In addition, the forces of capital and commerce blur for people a clean delineation of their needs as individuals and the needs which are socially constructed for us. People are expected and encouraged to choose socially acceptable alternatives. Choices are impinged upon by ideological constructions; for example, the pressure to be mothers. It is very difficult for women during pregnancy and birth, for example, to resist the use of new technologies. They can be accused of being selfish, of not thinking of the child first. The 'maternal' consciousness is shaped to be responsive to these arguments.

Proponents of technological intervention argue that informed consent to certain procedures is all that is necessary to ensure that choice has been exercised. But we could ask how well 'informed' the users of IVF are as to failure rates, for example, or the side effects of superovulation drugs. Are they told that some procedures are experimental, not therapeutic?

There is a difference between merely being issued information and discussing or negotiating the pros and cons of a procedure. For example, in one study, only half of the families given genetic counselling had actually grasped its impact.[14] Moreover, people can hardly exercise freedom of choice when hospitalised, frightened and/or in pain. They often relinquish power to the person who may heal them or solve their problems.

In his analysis of an example of medical experimentation without social accountability, George Annas looks at the 'Baby Fae' case where the heart of a baboon was transplanted into a newborn baby. Annas shows that consent was not based on adequate information in this case and that the Nuremberg Code was violated, as was the necessary prerequisite for human experimentation, that there be sufficient prior animal experimentation. Nor have IVF procedures been tested on primates first.[15] A federal ethics board in the United States of America in 1979, which held hearings on IVF, noted that there had been insufficient controlled animal research designed to determine the long-range effects of in vitro fertilisation and embryo transfer.[16] The board commented that this was noteworthy because there were available primate models (the 'models' now being used, of course, are women). Though the doctrine of informed consent has been operating for over twenty years in the US, doctors are failing to fulfil it. 'Failure to inform' has been behind the bulk of all 'wrongful birth' lawsuits.[17]

The informed consent debate places a great deal of faith in the individual's ability to make choices, in the doctor's beneficence and in patient autonomy. But as Janice Raymond has written, it

> seldom addresses the context in which choices are made, the patients' motivation to choose in certain ways, and the conditions that are necessary for a genuine autonomy to be exercised in the informed consent process.[18]

Few women in Western societies have the confidence to go through pregnancy and delivery without placing themselves in the hands of the technodocs; they regard most of the technologies used as 'routine'. As reproductive technology increases medical control of birth, pregnancy and now conception, and as pre-implantation diagnosis takes a hold, women learn to accept more and more intervention as 'routine'. Then the question of choice never arises. Barbara Katz Rothman writes:

> People do not need well-thought-out answers for why they do the accepted, expected thing. It is rather like asking someone why they wash their hands. The only necessary answer is 'because they get dirty'. It is self-evident, and does not warrant a discussion of the meaning of dirt or the value of cleanliness. Hands get washed when they are dirty; amnio gets done when you are over 35. It is routine.[19]

No one questions the need for routine amniocentesis. No one questions the routine use of ultrasound. Soon no one will question the routine screening of embryos before they are implanted.

In her discussion with Gena Corea on the developing surrogate motherhood industry, Andrea Dworkin addressed the concept of free will. Dworkin argues that the will is created outside the individual, influenced by social and economic factors; that individuality and free will are fictions for women because women are defined and used as a sex class. Dworkin notes

> the bitter fact that the only time that equality is considered a value in this society is in a situation like this where some extremely degrading transaction is being rationalized. And the only time that freedom is considered important to women as such is when we're talking

about the freedom to prostitute oneself in one way or another.[20]

'A WOMAN'S RIGHT TO CHOOSE'

In the social context of the values of individualism and liberalism, women in the women's movement were smart to develop the slogan 'a woman's right to choose'. It basically emerged in the late 1960s and early 1970s, a time when the women's movement was part of a general push by liberationist groups internationally.

A woman's right to choose has been linked primarily to the fight for access to safe abortion. Since the late 1970s when poor and minority women criticised the notion of 'choice', we have had to reassess its applicability. We can question whether the right to choose has been genuinely exercised if a woman aborts a female fetus because of the greater value her society puts on sons, if she aborts a Down's syndrome child because our society does not supply support for the raising of special-needs children, or aborts a wanted pregnancy because she is economically unable to support a child. In all these situations the notion of 'free' individual choice fails.

The new reproductive technologies too are producing scenarios which make slogans like 'a right to choose' simplistic in their practical application. In her discussions with women who underwent amniocentesis, Barbara Katz Rothman talks about their feeling that it was 'my only choice'. This, she says, occurs because the choices given to women are so negative that they take the way out which is least destructive for themselves and those around them. In such instances 'choice' is imposed upon the woman. This is particularly true with the new technologies of pre-natal assessment and 'selective reduction' (abortion). As Katz Rothman concludes:

> With birth control and abortion, women were able to choose not to bear children, not to be mothers. But with selective abortion, we ask mothers to decide just what kind of child they choose to mother. So choice enters a new arena of women's lives. In a world that supports and values neither mothers nor children, we ask individual mothers to look at their individual fetuses, and decide whether this child will be asking too much of her.[21]

Susan Himmelweit asserts that we need a broader basis on which to argue for access to abortion. She names that as humanitarian grounds, which she sees as a more secure basis for the availability of abortion than the rhetoric of choice. She writes:

> a mother before birth... may decide, for good reasons or bad, not to continue to nurture that child. If she does so, then a medical abortion is the safest way for her to proceed. To deny her that opportunity is therefore to risk her health and possibly her life; the alternative that she continues unwillingly to allow the foetus to grow within her is effectively enforcing her participation in a process that, like all nurturing, cannot be properly carried out by the unwilling. Some women in these circumstances may come to care for their foetus, as women have done with unwanted children, but the principle is the same. It is cruel to the unwanted foetus, just like an unwanted child, to enforce it upon an unwilling mother, and it is a singularly cruel punishment to impose upon the woman.[22]

We can support the availability of abortion on demand while still regretting that women may use abortion to abort female fetuses or disabled children. We need to work to maintain this access while creating a society in which such decisions need not be made so often, for as Himmelweit writes:

> Thus, another problem with the 'right to choose' is that the choices made by individuals may have social effects which are undesirable. Not only are individual's choices always made within an economic, cultural and political context, but that context is itself affected by the decisions of individuals.[23]

We need to question our attitudes to the disabled which the availability of abortion encourages us to gloss over. The attitude that a disabled person would be better eliminated may mean that the life of those who are disabled becomes more and more unpleasant as they become both fewer in number and are seen as 'failures' on the part of their mothers. Decisions to abort disabled or 'wrong-sex' fetuses feed into and continue to support the circumstances and attitudes which shaped that decision in the first place.

I have argued elsewhere that what feminists really mean by 'a woman's right to choose' is 'a woman's right to *control*'. Women claim the right to bodily integrity, to autonomy and to respect as moral human beings capable of making difficult decisions in this area. Women need access to abortion in order to control their lives in a less than perfect world. We have to ask the same question with respect to reproductive technology: does it necessarily increase the control of women over their lives? This book shows that it does not.

CONTROL AND THE NATURE OF POWER

The new reproductive technologies are controlled by those powerful groups who determine so much about our society, particularly the owners of information and technology. The state has some control through legislation over the progress or otherwise of science, science has control over its ethics and practice; but ultimately control in this field is exercised by the enormous multinational owners of the technology. Even in 1986, concern was expressed about the way genetic engineering was becoming a tool of insurance companies in the US. Multinational companies were looking at using genetic tests of workers' blood or urine, which could reveal markers of chromosomal susceptibility to various diseases and problems, in order to screen workers. McLoughlin wrote that

> Already, for instance, genetic screening can technically reveal an inherited tendency to develop a brain degenerative disease called Huntington's Chorea in middle age. Does a company hold back on investment in a young high-flyer once this risk is revealed in the genetic screening?

There was also concern raised by the trades unions that employers might cut corners on health and safety if they knew that they had workers who were already vulnerable to damage. Or

> technically, the employer could pick only workers with a genetic susceptibility to deafness, and when the worker is made deaf by the noise of the factory, avoid compensation by arguing that the worker would go deaf anyway.[24]

These technologies increase control by the powerful over those with less power. We are told that we will soon be able to control the quality of children; but we have to question who would set the control guidelines and how they would be implemented. Indeed, we have to ask why we would want to do such a thing. Barbara Katz Rothman wrote: 'it seems that, in gaining the choice to control the quality of our children, we may be losing the choice *not* to control the quality, the choice of simply accepting them as they are'.[25]

We cannot control the problem of less-than-perfect people by making disability 'an individual trouble', then telling a woman she has a choice when she makes the decision to abort a fetus with spina bifida if she lives in a fourth-floor apartment with no wheelchair access. In our society if you have a special-needs child you cannot even afford to die because society takes so little care of those who are not the perfect product. The social burden of people who are in special need is not shared equitably. But with the increasing development of these technologies, women will be accused of burdening society with less-than-perfect children if they go ahead and refuse technology. And as this increasingly becomes so, those who are born with a problem, or those who develop problems *after* birth (the majority of special-needs people) will be more and more disadvantaged as society develops a consciousness which says they should have been screened out in the first place.

Because many successful commercial enterprises are multinational, the implications for Third World women and communities are enormous. There is, for example, the possibility of enforced sterilisation of women, followed by IVF for those who are chosen as ideal breeders; coerced abortion for sex-selection purposes; and the traffic in children and women. Third World women themselves are constantly speaking out against the inter-relationship between the old and the new reproductive technologies, between sterilisation of women and their use of IVF, making the links with capital exploitation of the Third World by industrialised countries. In March 1989, the Feminist International Network of Resistance to Reproductive and Genetic Engineering (FINRRAGE) held an international conference in Bangladesh. One hundred and forty-five participants from thirty-five countries, mainly women from so-called 'developing' countries, discussed enforced sterilisation, the dumping of contraceptives on the Third

World and IVF as part of a population control programme. The use of sex selection to pick out female fetuses was also documented: women in poor countries are encouraged to sell their children even before birth. This has been occurring in India and in Bangladesh. One participant from Sri Lanka talked about the baby farms established there where pregnant women after birth immediately give their babies supposedly for intercountry adoption. At the end of the conference, participants drew up the Comilla Declaration, including the following statement:

> Having shared each other's experiences, insights, and knowledge, we women at the Bangladesh Conference reaffirmed our deep commitment to continue and intensify our work towards a humane and just world for all. We appeal to all women and men to unite globally against dehumanizing technologies and express solidarity with all those who seek to uphold and preserve the diversity of life on our planet and the integrity and dignity of all women.[26]

The control of conception is being taken over by laboratory technicians; women's control at the social and individual level is weakening. In 1990, a method was developed by which ovaries might be created from a fetus. Roger Gosden, the physiologist who made the discovery, said that 'the best source for human follicles would be the prenatal ovary'.[27] Ovaries, uteri which are functioning or created without women: what does this say of the integrity of the whole woman?

The ultimate control would of course be ectogenesis, life developed totally outside the womb, which Carlo Bulletti and his colleagues are working towards: their study was undertaken 'because future complete ectogenesis should not be ruled out'.[28] They have been working on maintaining uteri extracted from women outside of a woman's body.

As indicated earlier they have even implanted embryos into these wombs. Bongso in Singapore has also generated embryos in a woman's extracted womb lining (see Chapter 1). At Stanford University, scientists developed an artificial womb or fetal incubator. Oxygen and nutrients were pumped into it, and human fetuses which were products of spontaneous abortion have been kept alive for up to forty-eight hours.[29]

From the birth end of the continuum of pregnancy, younger and younger premature babies are kept alive in increasingly sophisticated artificial environments, possibly from twenty-four weeks. If we consider the process from the other end, that is from the point where an embryo is created in vitro, it is possible to keep them alive at least until the fourteenth day. If an artificial placenta could be perfected to bridge the time gap, an egg could be fertilised and brought to term within an artificial or 'glass womb'.[30] Development of the artificial womb has been promoted as having the following advantages: fetal medicine would be improved; the child could be immunised while still inside the 'womb'; geneticists could programme in some superior trait on which society would agree; sex determination would be simple; women would be spared the discomfort of childbirth; women could be permanently sterilised; and finally a man would be able to prove beyond a doubt that he is the father of the child.[31]

Male control could also come through the introduction of male 'mothers', men themselves bearing children. Though it seems fanciful, the precedents are there. In May 1979, a New Zealand woman, Margret Martin, gave birth to a baby girl having undergone a hysterectomy eight months earlier. The fertilised egg had lodged on her bowel, where it received enough nutrients to grow to term without the aid of a uterus. In about 1000 known cases a fertilised egg has worked its way into the abdominal cavity of a woman which can expand to accommodate the fetus. Approximately 9 per cent of these women have actually given birth to healthy children. The mother runs an enormous risk during this process and can often die from a massive haemorrhage. Dr Roy Hertz has had success with transplanting the eggs of a female baboon into the abdominal cavity of a male baboon, though he did not bring the fetus to term.[32] It appears that a fetus may be able to attach itself to any site which is rich in blood and nutrients.

The possibility of implanting a fertilised egg in the human male abdominal cavity has been discussed. A 'Linc' ('living' + 'incubator') pregnancy would involve the administration of hormones to the 'male mother' to 'mimic that of a pregnant woman', and delivering the baby through a laparotomy. It has also been suggested that a fertilised egg could be flushed out of a woman's womb and implanted into the man. As Dr Jules Black, a Fellow of the Royal Australian College of Obstetricians and Gynecologists, is reported as saying: 'This is the next step in in vitro fertilisation technology'.[33] Dr Alan Trounson, of the Monash IVF programme, reportedly saw no problem with male pregnancy: 'I think it is a challenge to women's roles but then women have challenged men's roles in the community. I don't see it as something we should be frightened of'.[34]

In recent years in Australia at least six popular magazines and newspapers have carried stories claiming transsexuals' 'right' to have children on IVF programmes. By July 1984 at least six male-to-female transsexuals had requested admittance to the IVF programme at the Queen Victoria Medical Centre.[35] There were suggestions that they could have their sperm frozen before the conversion operation and use a donor egg with their own sperm. They would then be both mother and father to the child. Dr Shettles, who has done pioneering work on IVF, commented: 'I don't think it's going to take as long as it did with the in vitro program. I think anyone who really wanted to get on with it now could achieve success'.[36] Published interviews with transsexuals who want to be involved in these kinds of programmes are constantly reappearing, indicating the beginning of 'softening up' the public to the idea before attempting it. Leaning on a rights-based argument, what they claim is their desire to be fulfilled within a stereotypic definition of femininity. As one article said, 'Phillip McKernan wants to give birth to prove something to himself—that he has finally made it as a woman'.[37] In a 1986 article, transsexual Estelle Croot said:

> I am a woman. And like any woman I want to feel complete, I want to be fulfilled and for me that means having a baby. I can't believe that the majority of Australians don't want me to have a baby.[38]

Professor William Walters, at that time a member of both the Monash IVF team and director of the Transsexual Conversion Clinic in Melbourne, said it is a '*natural corollary* (my emphasis) that they should want to have children'.[39]

Janice Raymond has argued convincingly that transsexualism represents the final colonisation of women.[40] Through a male-to-constructed-female sex change men are able to possess women's bodies, women's creative energies and women's capacities. These are the most feminine women: woman made by man to be as feminine as man deems fit. And now the man-made woman could become both mother and father to a child—the patriarchal dream/myth becomes reality.

Children then might be created that are neither borne by nor born of woman.

A gradual softening-up process to get the public to accept these technologies continues, with continuing discussions in the medical and ethical literature. It takes a great amount of emotional and intellectual strength to step back and see the processes which are going on around us. Discussing the inevitability of ectogenesis, Laurence Karp writes:

> The usual stepwise nature of medical and social progress probably will prevail: preliminary experimentation will lead to clinical use on a limited scale, which, in turn will generate further data. By the time the expanded clinical use comes under serious consideration, the public will have had time to assimilate the concepts involved, thereby dispelling the novelty and disposing of the initial horror. All things in good time.[41]

These developments would have seemed impossible and unbelievable ten years ago. Like Mary Shelley's book, *Frankenstein*, it shows how strong the desire is in man to be the creator to rival God and women in the control and creation of human life, and to determine what kind of life thrives.

Women do not control these processes. And if they did have access to control, they could not purify the technology out of its political base. They could not make the technology itself somehow benign. The technology and the purpose for its development are interdependent, perfectly co-joined. Lynda Lange summed up the reality of the situation for women when she wrote:

> Regardless of what may be technologically possible in the future, it seems unlikely that a technological approach will be any more useful for women than it has been for the elimination of such things as pollution, world hunger, etc. We have had the technology to solve these problems for some time, but politics and the imbalance of economic power have so far prevented this. The issues for women, as for everyone else, are not what we can do in principle (which changes constantly in unpredictable ways) but who is in control of what we can do.[42]

COLLUSION

In order to create resistance to this scientific vision of human society it is necessary to understand how science pushes ahead and is developing such a stranglehold on the direction of developments. Many aspects have been covered here: commercial forces and the scientific ethic based in patriarchal values; the ideologies which define motherhood as mandatory and the 'good woman' as inept socially and imperfect physically; an unthinking acceptance of technology as progress and a failure to analyse the commodification of life which is in progress around us; and finally, a tendency to resort to an easy individualism and liberalism which naively claims rights for people without considering the social implications.

There are women who lobby for reproductive and genetic engineering though they often want to extract and use IVF, while excluding other technologies, an impossible feat. Many support the technology because they want their suffering to have some meaning. It may, in their terms, help others if that suffering is used in some way by the technodocs. The reasons for women's collusion in such self-destructive programmes are complex. Desire, as already indicated, plays a large part. And this desire may be for a child or it may be a desire to resist the negative definitions of woman as invisible. The need to feel alive, to be noticed, central and visible is a powerful and understandable motivation. And the consciousness of women themselves is involved here. We are all products of ideology and express that influence differently. The ideology of motherhood and the good woman are powerful and difficult to resist. In the chapters on surrogacy and IVF, women themselves express this influence.

The nature of power differences between women and men means that at a consciousness level, women are constantly developing strategies for survival. Power often enforces psychological submission which can also lead in Kate Millett's terms to 'a kind of psychological addiction to self-denigration'.[43] Women need to believe in the benevolent nature of men and of medicine, into whose hands they place so much of themselves. Discussing the fate of the powerless and powerful, Wrong describes the experience thus:

> Helpless to resist coercion, fearful of punishment, dependent on the powerful for satisfaction of basic needs and for any opportunities for autonomous choice and activity, the powerless are inescapably subject to a will to believe in the ultimate benevolence of the power holder, in his acceptance in the last analysis of some limits to what he will demand of or inflict upon them, grounded in at least a residual concern for their interests.[44]

And the less powerful judge where their best chances lie. It is often the case that 'the powerless are not quick to put their faith in the powerless. The powerless need the powerful'.[45]

Women collude with medical science because they want a sense of control and hope that this is a way of obtaining it. Frances Evans analysed the inductions performed in Britain: these had increased from 14 per cent in 1963 to 41 per cent in 1974 as a proportion of total deliveries. The women concerned felt humiliated and indignant throughout the processes of pregnancy, felt they had minimal control over the care they were receiving and were dissatisfied with the way the care was delivered, yet they still had faith in the medical profession. They expressed a contradictory wish for more control over their pregnancies alongside the push for a greater use of technology, which would mean yielding control to technicians. Evans concludes: 'it now seems that this is not so much a contradiction as two sides of the same coin: that of women's uncertainty and ignorance, fostered by the male monopoly of medical knowledge and decision making'.[46]

Catherine Kohler Riessman has argued that women have actively collaborated in an increased medicalisation of their lives, starting with childbirth in the eighteenth and nineteenth centuries. They did this for a complex set of reasons. Among them was fear, as women from all classes experienced birth as terrifying. They also wanted relief from pain and this led to the development of anaesthesia in childbirth. Childbirth itself was a dangerous business and women became convinced by the medical profession that they needed increased technological intervention to have safer birth. This allowed physicians to gain control of the market, including routine births in which there were no problems. It introduced a distance between women and their bodies during birth, beginning the process of the alienation of women from reproduction.

Women also pushed for increased control in contraception but ended up with a dangerous high-technology 'solution'. There are times when the interests of women are served by the medical profession whose political and economic interests are in turn served by turning women's problems into illnesses. Women desire the acknowledgement of medicine that their experience is valid, and medicine responds by medicalising it.[47] Throughout this process, women are gradually relinquishing control.

A similar analysis can be conducted on reproductive technology. Here there is a socially constructed desire expressed by one group of women which has been taken up and validated by the medical profession for its own purposes. Medicos then introduce a technology based on this desire for the production of drugs and specific technological implements. They even sell their expertise. Throughout this process women scramble to maintain control. Although constrained, as we all are, by ideological beliefs and assumptions and by the power structures operating in society, the women on IVF programmes themselves are maintaining a resistance to the encroachment of medicine. The active campaign of some women with respect to policy-making and the improving of conditions for users of IVF is evidence of this. But these attempts to improve conditions do nothing to change the material, social and ideological conditions in which the relationship between medicine, commerce and consciousness is taking place.

The collusion of some women in the progress of medical technology is a complicated relationship based in their political belief about personal control. Activism within this collusion means women have changed some of the negative experiences which, for example, women on IVF have registered. Resistance, then, occurs from women within research programmes, as well as from women outside them fighting for their termination. The role of woman as victim and resister is complex.

RESISTANCE

There have always been some women who have expressed resistance to patriarchy. Those who work in the paid worforce already undermine the current definition of motherhood with its essential economic dependence on a man, even though they do not often gain equal power through their paid labour. Single heterosexual women who mother outside of the control of marriage also express resistance to the motherhood myth. So too do lesbian mothers, whether they come from heterosexual marriages or establish families of their own.

For those who want to resist the kind of world into which science is ignorantly leading us, what forms of action are open which could challenge, impede or even stop it?

At the individual level the minds and consciousness of women need to be changed. It is crucial to empower women with a sense of disbelief about the negative self-definitions which have been created for them. Women need to be empowered with a sense of self full of the dignity and integrity which are essential to political action. No revolutionary change comes from those who believe their oppression is justified or who do not recognise it.

Women need to reject the equation of personhood with fertility. It is difficult to know how many infertile women resist technology, though there is evidence in the growing number of self-help groups outside the medical system that this is inceasing. Many of the women who have used the technology and have withdrawn from it gain a great deal in self-knowledge. Isabelle Bainbridge felt that after seventeen years of attempting to have a child 'coming to terms with infertility and learning to live past it has challenged my life in a way which no pregnancy or child could ever have done for me'.[48] Bainbridge had seven IVF treatments which she described as 'a very brutal way' of coming to terms with infertility. She eventually left the programme to counsel other women, to assist them with the grief of infertility, claiming that there are other ways in which a woman can use 'mothering instincts'.

Women repeatedly say that the more the technologies become available the harder it is to give up the concept of biological womanhood. Yet in Lasker and Borg's study more than a third of the women had rejected the idea of IVF because of poor success rates and the brutality of treatment. They quote one woman who decided to stop treatment and who expressed her enormous relief:

> I knew that there was a point when I had to quit. There are just so many times I could allow this kind of invasion, not only into my body, but into my psyche.

> I don't know how long you can hang onto the word *hopeful.* You have to come to a time when you say it's over. It was such a relief to put it behind me and get on with my life.[49]

The development of self-help groups to assist women to find other ways of dealing with their infertility has been an important new move. The group in Perth, Western Australia, for example, Issues (In) Fertility, has had enormous success in either assisting women to become pregnant by other non-invasive methods or in moving away from the trauma of infertility on to the next stage of their lives. Infertile feminist women have been developing counselling strategies and centres for infertile women. Some of these developments are documented in Renate Klein's book *Infertility*. As Klein writes,

> No matter how clear the danger of the technology is, this alone may not be enough to convince women who think they must 'try everything' not to use them. In addition to warnings against the technologies, what we must also provide are *visions* for a different kind of life: a life without one's own biological children perhaps, a life in which a woman is valued for herself, a life in which women value themselves. This entails nothing less than working towards a society that cherishes a woman's full humanity as an invaluable part of the community; that sees her as a whole person and not as a female incubator destined to give birth. Fertile and infertile we can all help to de-stigmatise infertility, to remove those feelings of shame, worthlessness and despair of which we have heard many times...

These arguments are not a judgement against women who want to use the technology. Feminism is a politics that attacks 'the institutions and the powerful, not the individual women'.[50] When all the influences that operate upon women are considered, it is understandable that some strive to fulfil their socially required role. What is not acceptable is that they do this in a manner which is self-abusive; they should not be supported if they place feminist principles and women as a social group at risk of losing control of procreation. But it is not women who are the problem; the problem lies in patriarchal structures and patriarchal ideology. In her analysis of prostitution, Carole Pateman makes the same point when she argues that the criticism of prostitution…

> is likely to provoke the accusation that contemporary contractarians [libertarians] bring against feminists, that criticism of prostitution shows contempt for prostitutes. To argue that there is something wrong with prostitution does not necessarily imply any adverse judgement on the women who engage in the work. When socialists criticize capitalism and the employment contract they do not do so because they are contemptuous of workers, but because they are the workers' champions.[51]

At the social level resistance comes through giving voice to women who have rejected technology or who have learned different ways of dealing with infertility. It comes from people becoming more articulate on the issues involved. The evidence should be made accessible so that the community understands what science is doing. There needs to be political activism for preventative medicine, and political activism for the establishment of law.

The Feminist International Network of Resistance to Reproductive and Genetic Engineering (FINRRAGE) is active in these ways. Created in 1984, with members currently in forty countries, it has developed four main strategies for creating change in this area: the exchange of information and the development of activism; the development of research into the field to create feminist theory and practice; the publication of such information and research to make it more accessible to a wider audience; pressure tactics through the media and lobbying to influence legislation and social debate.

The exchange of information has led to the development of a self-funding network into which members feed readings from journals and newspapers. These, along with information on activism by members, are sent to an international co-ordinator who circulates packages to the national co-ordinators. Information is also exchanged at conferences arranged for activists only, to date in Sweden, Belgium, Britain, Australia, Bangladesh, Germany, Spain and Brazil. This grassroots work also involves speaking to general-interest and professional groups on the work of members and on the latest developments in reproductive and genetic engineering. Members are also involved in creating feminist theory (and therefore practice) around these technologies, publishing the results.[52]

Finally, members have been active lobbyists for legislative change, using the media, pressure groups and direct approaches to parliamentarians. Gena Corea and Janice Raymond helped to establish the National Coalition Against Surrogacy in the United States of America which included in its membership a considerable number of past 'surrogates', and they have given testimony to various US Senate hearings. Australian members have also regularly appeared as witnesses at government hearings.[53] Australian feminists have also been particularly successful in their media work, bringing the feminist position directly to the public through the press.

One of the issues that many members in FINRRAGE have pursued is that of legislation. It is essential that people become informed about the laws concerning reproductive and genetic engineering. Government committees often call for public submissions on issues and it is important that members of the community respond. There are of course dangers in the development of legislation, as it can be and often is used against women. In the field of reproductive technology, legislation is often embryo-centred and not woman-centred.

The difficulty here is that without law this field of work will continue totally unregulated. The experimentation on women has the possibility of being even more brutal than it would be without the control of legislation. The law can in fact stop some research from taking place. In the states of Victoria, South Australia and Western Australia, and in British legislation, the cloning of human beings and the inauguration of trans-species work with humans (the implantation of animal material into humans and vice versa) is not allowed. Surrogacy will be illegal in all Australian states soon. Embryo experimentation is banned or controlled in most states.

Ultimately laws will be made, and women need to be a part of that process. They should push for stopping reproductive technology, not regulating it; regulation implies acceptance of the technology under certain guidelines. The alternative of no legislation is a totally free market which exploits women more, particularly less powerful women.

Scientists, in comparison, feel they are a law unto themselves. Although they profess that they are seeking community debate, when the community creates legislation to control their work they actively work against it. They claim the ability to self-regulate, yet the evidence of their actions does not support their rhetoric. Where there is so much profit to be made, medical researchers cannot be the guardians of ethical values. Unless the community attempts to take control through legislation, medical research in association with commercial interests will be determining the nature of our society.

My own basis for opposing the current path of this technology rests in the feminist moral values outlined above. By this I do not mean an empty moralism, 'a set of rules learned by rote that keeps women locked in... a defense against experiencing the world'.[54] Rather, feminism for me is a political and social theory based in what Andrea Dworkin calls a moral intelligence.

> Moral intelligence demands a nearly endless exercise of the ability to make decisions: significant decisions; decisions inside history, not peripheral to it; decisions about the meaning of life; decisions that arise from an acute awareness of one's own mortality.[55]

It is the obligation of agents of social change to look beyond the self and engage in this moral activity. This often means coming up against painful decisions. It also requires moral imagination, to develop a vision of what we would like our society to be. Succumbing half-heartedly to the belief that social change is too difficult and that technology will over-run us after all is a negative way of living; whereas feminism is an activist, and optimistic, philosophy. It looks for the good in people. It seeks to construct a society in which there is fulfilment for individuals, balanced with a reciprocal responsibility to the social group. Most importantly it concentrates on *relationships* between people. If we forget that people, primarily women and children, are involved in these technological experiments, we call into question our human obligations. And this is profoundly unethical.

In our society today there is an opportunity to stop the movement which is occurring towards the dehumanisation and commodification of living beings. It is possible to stop the processes which are turning women into living laboratories and children into products for sale or exchange. Though they are not always articulate and though they are not always heard, there are many who share the desire for a more humane vision of the future. A unification of that purpose, a belief in the possibility for change and a concern for the generations coming after, should be a solid base from which to counter the thoughtless pursuit of scientific control and the greed for profit which current reproductive and genetic engineering represent.

NOTES AND REFERENCES

INTRODUCTION

1 Gena Corea, What the King cannot see, paper delivered to the Law Reform Commission of Victoria, May 1986, pp. 16–17.
2 Interview with Dr Max Brinsmead by Calvin Miller, 'When a foetus is a "Mother"', *Australian Doctor Weekly*, 27 May 1988.
3 Bob Dvorchak, 'Surrogate mothers: Pregnant idea now a pregnant business', *Los Angeles Herald Examiner*, 27 December 1983, p. A1.
4 Herbert F. Krimmel, 'The Case Against Surrogate Parenting', in Carol Levine (ed.), *Taking Sides: Clashing Views on Controversial Bio-Ethical Issues*, Dushkin, Guildford, Connecticut, 1984.
5 The term 'control myth' is Elizabeth Janeway's; see *Powers of the Weak*, Knopf, New York, 1980.
6 Mary Shelley, *Frankenstein or the Modern Prometheus*, edited by M.K. Joseph, Oxford University Press, Oxford, 1969, pp. 54, 140.
7 Carole Pateman, *The Sexual Contract*, Polity Press, Oxford, 1988, p. 19.
8 Witness the bestowal or withdrawal of public child care and the chequered history of maternity leave.
9 It should be remembered that patriarchal control through force can operate at the state, social and individual level, through argument, rape, incest, battery or the violence of pornography. The knowledge of male violence creates a culture of terrorism. This is not too strong a definition when women live with the knowledge that the majority of violence towards them takes place within the 'haven' of the home and where women are more frequently raped by men they know and are connected with than by men they do not.
10 Barbara Ehrenreich, and Deirdre English, *For Her Own Good: 150 Years of the Experts' Advice to Women*, Doubleday, New York, 1979.
11 Elizabeth W. Moen, 'What Does "Control Over Our Bodies" Really Mean?', *International Journal of Women's Studies* 2, 1979, pp. 129–43.
12 Nancy Folbre, 'Of patriarchy born: the political economy of fertility decisions', *Feminist Studies* 9, 2, 1983, pp. 261–84.
13 Judith Lorber, 'Considering a biosocial perspective on parenting', *Signs. Journal of Women in Culture and Society* 4, 4, 1979, pp. 701–3.
14 Joanne Finkelstein, and Patricia Clough, 'Foetal politics and the birthof an industry', *Women's Studies International Forum* 6, 4, 1983, p. 396.

15 Eva Feder Kittay, 'Womb envy: an explanatory concept', in Joyce Trebilcot (ed.), *Mothering. Essays in feminist theory*, Rowman & Allanheld, New Jersey, 1984, pp. 94–128.
16 Finkelstein and Clough, p. 396.
17 Mary O'Brien, *The Politics of Reproduction*, Routledge & Kegan Paul, London, 1981, pp. 33–4.
18 Pateman, p. 35.
19 O'Brien, p. 46.
20 Azizah al-Hibri, 'Reproduction, mothering and the origins of patriarchy', in Trebilcot, pp. 85–6.
21 Pateman, p. 214.
22 Pateman, p. 215.
23 Pateman, p. 216.

1. IN VITRO FERTILISATION: MAN MAKES THE EMBRYO

1 Fiona Whitlock, 'Australia's IVF teams lead the world', *Weekend Australian Magazine*, 17–18 August 1985, p. 6.
2 Louise Carbines, 'Pregnant—with egg from another woman', *Age*, 12 March 1983, p. 1.; 'The tragedy behind two frozen embryos', *New Idea*, 4 August 1984, pp. 32–4; Nene King and Jo Wiles, 'These little girls are twins ... born 18 months apart', *New Idea*, 26 October 1985, pp. 8–11; 'The frozen embryo baby: Zoe, you're a world first', *New Idea*, 21 April 1984, pp. 3–9; Jo Wiles, 'Margaret, giving birth to a miracle', *New Idea*, 19 May 1984, pp. 4–5; 'Test-tube quins born', *Age*, 31 March 1986; 'Hearty twins hailed as in vitro victory,' *Age*, 5 July 1986; '"Frozen" baby No. 4'. *Geelong Advertiser*, 29 October 1984; 'Our babies are still world-beaters', *New Idea*, 22 March 1986, pp. 18–19; 'Amy is 18 months old. Her twin sister was born on Tuesday', *Herald*, 23 April 1987; 'Embrionic first', *Australian*, 26 February 1988; 'New test tube techniques produce "first" pregnancy', *Guardian*, 3 April 1989; 'Pregnancy for women with no ovaries', *Australian*, 7 August 1985, p. 5.
3 Renate Klein, *Exploitation of a desire. Women's experiences with in vitro fertilisation*, Women's Studies Summer Institute, Deakin University Press, Geelong, 1989, p. 30.
4 Renate Klein (ed.), *Infertility. Women speak out about their experiences of reproductive medicine*, Pandora Press, London, 1989.
5 Miriam D. Mazor, 'Barren couples', *Psychology Today* 12, 1979, pp. 103, 104.
6 Naomi Pfeffer, 'Artificial insemination and infertility', in Michelle Stanworth (ed.), *Reproductive Technologies: Gender, Motherhood and Medicine*, Polity Press, Cambridge, 1987, p. 86.
7 ibid., p. 87.
8 Naomi Pfeffer and Anne Woollett, *The Experience of Infertility*, Virago, London, 1983, p. 103.

9 ibid., p. 105.
10 Eileen Alderton, 'Infertility: A special report', *Australian Women's Weekly*, 28 July 1982, p. 65.
11 Katharina Stens, 'Give me children or else I die', in Klein, *Infertility*, p. 15.
12 Ioannis E. Messinis, Allan Templeton, Roslyn Angell and John Aitken, 'A Comparison of Fixed Regimens For Obtaining Human Cleaving Oocytes For Research Purposes', *British Journal of Obstetrics and Gynaecology* 93, 1986, pp. 39-42; Judith N. Lasker and Susan Borg, *In Search of Parenthood: Coping with Infertility and High-Tech Conception*, Beacon Press, Boston, 1987.
13 Cynthia Gorney, 'For love and money', *California Magazine*, October 1983, pp. 88-155; Klein, *Infertility*.
14 Michael Pirrie, 'New IVF treatment stopped', *Age*, 2 April 1988.
15 *Mims Annual*, IMS Publishing, Sydney, 1984, 1987.
16 Carole Dettmann and Douglas Saunders. *The Chance of a Lifetime: Infertility and IVF*, Penguin, Melbourne, p. 214; Pfeffer and Woollett.
17 Cited in Françoise Laborie, 'New reproductive technologies: News from France and elsewhere', *Reproductive and Genetic Engineering. Journal of International Feminist Analysis* 1, 1, 1988, p. 81.
18 R.N. Porter, W. Smith, I.L. Craft, N.A. Abdulwahid and H.S. Jacobs, 'Induction of ovulation for in vitro fertilisation using buserelin and gonadotropins', *Lancet*, 1 December 1984, p. 1285.
19 Anne Rochon Ford, 'Hormones: getting out of hand', in Kathleen McDonnell (ed.), *Adverse Effects: Women and the Pharmaceutical Industry*, The Women's Press, Toronto, 1986, p. 31.
20 Gena Corea, *The Mother Machine. From Artificial Insemination to Artificial Wombs*, Harper & Row, New York, 1985, p. 111.
21 Ana Regina Gomez dos Reis, 'IVF in Brazil: the story told by the newspapers', in Patricia Spallone and Deborah Lynn Steinberg (eds), *Made to Order: The Myth of Reproductive and Genetic Progress*, Pergamon Press, Oxford, 1987, p. 120-32; Anne Treweek, 'Unusual death of IVF patient', *West Australian*, 5 August 1987, p. 2; 'Perth IVF deaths', *FINRRAGE Newsletter* 1, 2, 1988, p. 2.
22 Wilfried Feichtinger and Peter Kemeter, 'Laparoscopic or ultrasonically guided follicle aspiration for in vitro fertilization?', *Journal of in Vitro Fertilization and Embryo Transfer* 1, 4, 1984, pp. 244-9.
23 Suzan Lenz, 'Ultrasonic-guided follicle puncture under local anesthesia', *Journal of in Vitro Fertilization and Embryo Transfer* 1, 4, 1984, pp. 239-43.
24 Joseph D. Schulman, 'Laparoscopy for in vitro fertilization: end of an era', *Fertility and Sterility* 44, 5, 1985.
25 Lenz, p. 240; Gena Corea and Susan Ince, 'IVF a game for losers at half of U.S. clinics', *Medical Tribune* 26, 19, 1985, pp. 11-13.
26 Lenz, pp. 240, 241.

27 ibid., p. 242.
28 P. Dellenbach, I. Nisand, L. Moreau, B. Feger, C. Plumere, P. Gerlinger, B. Brun and Y. Rumplen, 'Transvaginal sonigraphically controlled ovarian follicle puncture for egg retrieval', *Lancet*, 30 June 1984, p. 1467.
29 Schulman.
30 Feichtinger and Kemeter.
31 'Transvaginal oocyte retrieval called preferred method in IVF', *Ob.Gyn.News* 21, 22, 1986, pp. 2, 26.
32 'Laparoscopy may be best way to obtain oocytes', *Ob.Gyn.News* 20, 9, 1985, p. 38.
33 Schulman.
34 Klein, *Exploitation.*
35 Gena Corea and Susan Ince, 'Report of a survey of IVF clinics in the US', in Spallone and Steinberg p. 142.
36 ibid., p. 143.
37 Klein, *Exploitation*, p. 27.
38 Ronald C. Strickler, Cat Christianson, James P. Crane, Andi Curato, Alfred B. Knight and Victoria Yang, 'Ultrasound guidance for human embryo transfer', *Fertility and Sterility* 43, 1, 1985, pp. 54-61.
39 Phillip L. Matson, David C. Blackledge, Peter A. Richardson, Simon R. Turner, Jeanne M. Yovich and John L. Yovich, 'Pregnancies after pronuclear stage transfer', *Medical Journal of Australia* 146, 5 January 1987, p. 60.
40 Katie Ruddon, '400 couples in line for gamete intrafallopian transfer', *Ob.Gyn.News* 20, 4, 1985, p. 16.
41 'Intratubal insemination: alternative to intrafallopian transfer?' *Ob. Gyn.News* 23, 1, 1988, p. 51.
42 'Transutero-tubal insemination for poor semen quality', *Ob.Gyn. News* 22, 13, 1987, p. 9.
43 'Alternative to IVF and gamete intrafallopian transfer described', loc.cit.
44 'New alternatives to in-vitro fertilization assessed', *Ob.Gyn.News* 21, 12, 1986, p. 1.
45 David S. McLaughlin, Donald E. Troike, Thomas R. Tegenkamp and Donald G. McCarthy, 'Tubal ovum transfer: a catholic-approved alternative to in-vitro fertilisation', *Lancet*, January 24 1987, p. 214.
46 King and Wiles.
47 Calvin Miller, 'Frozen ova may help solve in vitro ethics dilemma', *Age*, 7 March 1985.
48 A. Bernard, D.A. Imoedemhe, R.W. Shaw and B. Fuller, 'Effects of cryoprotectants on human oocyte', *Lancet*, 16 March 1985, p. 632; Joan Phyland, 'Frozen egg technology could cause genetic defects, says IVF expert', *Advertiser*, 15 July 1986, p. 3; Matthew Warren, 'World's first births from frozen eggs', *Australian*, 5-6 July 1986, p. 1.

49 Phyland; Noel Rait, 'Frozen-egg twins make history', *New Idea*, 11 October 1986, pp. 10–11; Christopher Chen, 'Pregnancy after human oocyte preservation', *Lancet*, 19 April 1986, pp. 884–6.
50 'Oocyte donation, freezing found increasingly successful', *Ob.Gyn. News* 22, 12, 1987, pp. 2, 21.
51 Ann Pappert, 'New technology poses ethical dilemma', *Globe and Mail*, 9 February 1988, p. A18.
52 National Perinatal Statistics Unit, University of Sydney, 1990.
53 *In Vitro Fertilization in Australia*, Commonwealth Department of Community Services and Health, Canberra, 1988, p. 44.
54 Phyland.
55 'Doctor plans egg bank', *Geelong Advertiser*, 20 April 1988.
56 'Frozen eggs find ethical favour in Australia', *New Scientist*, 24 April 1986, p. 22.
57 Heather Carswell, 'See many unanswered questions on cryopreservation', *Ob.Gyn.News* 21, 23, 1986, p. 9.
58 ibid.
59 Judith N. Lasker and Susan Borg, *In Search of Parenthood: Coping With Infertility and High-Tech Conception*, Beacon Press, Boston, 1987.
60 M. Bustillo and J. Buste, 'Non-surgical ovum transfer as a treatment in infertile women', *Journal of the American Medical Association* 251, 9, 1984, pp. 1171–3; H. Jones, 'Variations on a theme' (editorial), *Journal of the American Medical Association* 250, 16, 1983, p. 2182–3.
61 L. Walters, 'Ethical aspects of surrogate embryo transfer' (editorial), *Journal of the American Medical Association* 250, 16, 1983, p. 2183.
62 Lasker and Borg, p. 94.
63 loc.cit.
64 Walters.
65 Lasker and Borg, p. 97.
66 'Several alternatives hold promise for infertile if IVF fails', *Ob.Gyn. News* 22, 2, 1987, p. 27.
67 Lasker and Borg, p. 96.
68 ibid., p. 101.
69 Sandra Blakeslee, 'Trying to make money making "test-tube" babies', *New York Times*, 17 May 1987, p. 6F.
70 'Uterine lavage, reimplantation yield pregnancy in 8 of 56 tries', *Ob.Gyn.News* 22, 10, 1987, p. 26.
71 Philip McIntosh, 'Research council rejects surrogate embryo transfer', *Age*, 22 February 1985.
72 Michael Pirrie, 'Hospital seeks egg donors', *Age*, 27 October 1989.
73 Andrea Laws-King, Alan Trounson, Henry Sathananthan and Ismail Kola, 'Fertilization of human oocytes by microinjection of a single spermatozoon under the zona pellucida', *Fertility and Sterility* 48, 4, 1987, pp. 637–42.

74 Sandra Lee, 'Scientist defends new IVF technique', *Herald*, 6 April 1988.
75 Richard Gluyas, 'Nature makes choice in chosen IVF technique', *Australian*, 8 April 1988.
76 Di Webster, 'IVF technique may raise success rate', *Sunday Age*, 9 September 1990.
77 'Intravaginal culture, embryo transfer could reduce cost of IVF', *Ob.Gyn.News* 22, 12, 1987, p. 30.
78 ibid.
79 Elizabeth Kane, *Birth Mother*, Sun Books, Melbourne, 1988.
80 'Commonwealth Perspectives on IVF Funding', Department of Community Services and Health, Canberra, 1988; *Age Good Weekend*, 31 March, 1991.
81 Ditta Bartels, The public costs of IVF programs, paper presented at the annual symposium of the Australian Academy of the Social Sciences, 11 November 1987, p. 85.
82 Klein, *Exploitation*; Christine Crowe, 'Women want it: in-vitro fertilization and women's motivations for participation', *Women's Studies International Forum* 8, 6, 1985, pp. 547-52.
83 Bartels.
84 *FINRRAGE Newsletter*, May 1988, p. 5.
85 Diagnosis Pty Ltd, *A Consultancy Report on IVF in Australia*, Department of Community Services and Health, Canberra, 1988, p. 14.
86 Bartels, p. 8.
87 'Commonwealth Perspectives on IVF Funding' (Summary), pp. 6-7.
88 Corea and Ince.
89 'In vitro fertilization/embryo transfer in the United States: 1985 and 1986 results from the National IVF/ET registry', *Fertility and Sterility* 49, 2, 1988, pp. 212-15.
90 Ann Pappert, 'Success rates quoted by in vitro clinics not what they seem', *Globe and Mail*, 8 February 1988, p. A3.
91 Diagnosis Pty Ltd, p. 35.
92 Michael R. Soules, 'The in vitro fertilization pregnancy rate: let's be honest with one another', *Fertility and Sterility* 43, 4, 1985, pp. 511-13.
93 Fiona J. Stanley, 'In vitro fertilisation—a GIFT for the infertile or a cycle of despair?', *Medical Journal of Australia* 148, 1988, pp. 15-19.
94 Bartels.
95 Diagnosis Pty Ltd, Table 6.
96 Chris Anne Raymond, 'In vitro fertilization enters stormy adolescence as experts debate the odds', *Journal of the American Medical Association* 259, 4, 1988, pp. 464-9.
97 'IVF and GIFT Pregnancies in Australia and New Zealand 1988', National Perinatal Statistics Unit (NPSU), Sydney, 1990.
98 'How many oocytes?', *Lancet*, 21 May 1988, p. 1178.
99 *Infertility*, Office of Technology Assessment, USA, 1988, p. 295.

100 Pappert, p. A3.
101 John A. Collins et al., 'Treatment-independent pregnancy among infertile couples', *New England Journal of Medicine* 309, 20, 1983, pp. 1201-6.
102 Z. Ben-Rafael, J. Dor, S. Mashiach, 'Treatment-independent pregnancy among patients following an in vitro fertilization and embryo transfer trial', *Journal of in Vitro Fertilization and Embryo Transfer* 1, 2, 1984, p. 99.
103 Cited in Chris Anne Raymond, p. 465.
104 'Difficulty in defining infertility confounds epidemiologic research', *Ob.Gyn.News* 22, 1, 1987, p. 13.
105 Pappert, p. A3.
106 This research is part of collaborative work undertaken with Dr Renate Klein: R. Klein/R. Rowland, 'Women as test sites for fertility drugs: clomiphene citrate and hormonal cocktails', *Reproductive and Genetic Engineering. Journal of International Feminist Analysis* 1, 3, 1988, pp. 251-73.
107 'IVF and GIFT Pregnancies... 1988'.
108 James H. Clark and Shirley McCormack, 'The effect of Clomid and Other Triphenylethylene Derivatives During Pregnancy and The Neonatal Period', *Journal of Steroid Biochemistry* 12, 1980, pp. 47-53.
109 Anita Direcks and Helen Bequaert Holmes, 'Miracle Drug, Miracle Baby', *New Scientist*, 6 November 1986, pp. 53-55.
110 Shirley G. Driscoll and Stephanie H. Taylor, 'Effects of Prenatal Maternal Estrogen on the Male Urogenital System', *Obstetrics and Gynecology* 56, 5, 1980, pp. 537-42.
111 Gena Corea, *The Hidden Malpractice: How American Medicine Mistreats Women*, Harper & Row, New York, 1985; Direcks and Holmes; Diana Scully, *Men Who Control Women's Health. The Miseducation of Obstetrician-Gynaecologists*, Houghton Mifflin, Boston, 1980; Driscoll and Taylor.
112 Anita Direcks and Ellen Hoen, 'The Crime Continues', McDonnell, pp. 41-50.
113 G.R. Cunha, O. Taguchi, R. Namikawa, Y. Nishizuka and S.J. Robbey, 'Teratogenic Effects of Clomiphene, Tamoxifen, and Diethylstilbestrol on the Developing Human Female Genital Tract', *Human Pathology* 18, 1987, pp. 1132-43.
114 James W. Newberne, William L. Kuhn and John R. Elsea, 'Toxicologic Studies on Clomiphene', *Toxicology and Applied Pharmacology* 9, 1966, pp. 44-56; James H. Clark and Shirley McCormack, 'Clomid or Nafoxidine Administered to Neonatal Rats Causes Reproductive Tract Abnormalities', *Science* 197, 1977, pp. 164-5. R.H. Gorwill, H.D. Steele and I.R. Sarda, 'The Effect of Clomiphene Citrate on the Developing Mouse Vagina', *Fertility and Sterility* 34, 2, 1980, p. 190.

115 *Mims Annual*, IMS Publishing, Sydney 1984, 1987.
116 W.D.A. Ford and K.E.T. Little, 'Fetal Ovarian Dysplasia Possibly Associated With Clomiphene', *Lancet*, 14 November 1981, p. 1107; I.A. Laing, C.R. Steer, J. Dudgeon and J.K. Brown, 'Clomiphene and Congenital Retinopathy', *Lancet*, 14 November 1981, pp. 1107-8.
117 Jennifer L. Dyson and H.G. Kohler, 'Anencephaly and Ovulation Stimulation', *Lancet*, 2 June 1973, pp. 1256-7.
118 Y. Biale, M. Leventhal, Altaras and N. Ben-Aderet, 'Anencephaly and Clomiphene-Induced Pregnancy', *Acta Obstet.Gynecol.Scand.* 57, 1978, pp. 483-4.
119 Paul A.L. Lancaster, 'Congenital Malformations after in-vitro fertilization', *Lancet*, December 1987, pp. 1392-3; Keiichi Kurachi, Toshihiro Ano, Junnosuke Minagawa, and Akira Miyake, 'Congenital Malformations of Newborn Infants After Clomiphene-Induced Ovulation', *Fertility and Sterility* 40, 2, 1983, pp. 187-9; Mars Ahlgren, Bengt Kallen and Gunnar Rannevik, 'Outcome of Pregnancy After Clomiphene Therapy', *Acta.Obstet.Gynecol.Scand.* 55, 1976, pp. 371-5.
120 Michelle Plachot, Anne-Marie Junca, Jacqueline Mandelbaum, J. de Grouchy, J. Salat-Baroux and J. Cohen, 'Chromosome Investigations in Early Life. I. Human Oocytes Recovered in an IVF Programme', *Human Reproduction* 1, 8, 1986, pp. 547-51; H. Wramsby and P. Liedholm, 'A Gradual Fixation Method For Chromosomal Preparations of Human Oocytes', *Fertility and Sterility* 41, 1984, pp. 736-8; Horst Spielman et al., 'Abnormal Chromosomal Behaviour in Human Oocytes Which Remained Unfertilized During Human In Vitro Fertilization', *Journal of in Vitro Fertilization and Embryo Transfer* 2, 3, 1985, pp. 138-42; Hakan Wramsby, Karl Fredga and Percy Liedholm, 'Chromosome Analysis of Human Oocytes Recovered From Preovulatory Follicles in Stimulated Cycles', *New England Journal of Medicine* 316, 3, 1987, pp. 121-4.
121 'Offspring don't seem to be at a risk from ovulation inducing drugs', *Ob.Gyn.News* 22, 7, 1987, p. 6.
122 Barbara Field and Charles Kerr, 'Ovulation Stimulation and Defects of Neural Tube Closure', *Lancet*, 21 December 1974, p. 1511.
123 Philip McIntosh, 'Birth defects claim fuels campaign against IVF', *Age*, 8 January 1988.
124 *Mims Annual*, 1987, p. 373.
125 Dorothy Lipovenko, 'Fertility Drug Causes Tissue Changes in Mice, MD Says', *Globe and Mail*, 14 May 1984, p. 3; Ford and Little, p. 1107.
126 Cunha et al., p. 1142.
127 Ford and Little, p.1107.
128 Ann Pappert, 'Critics Worry Women Not Told of Fertilisation Program Risks', *Globe and Mail*, 6 February 1988, p. 14.

129 Gabor T. Kovacs, Peter M. Dennis, Rhonda J. Shelton, Ken H. Outch, Robert A. McLean, David L. Healy and Henry G. Burger, 'Induction of Ovulation with Human Pituitary Gonadotrophin', *Medical Journal of Australia*, 12 May 1984, pp. 575-9; A. Birkenfeld et al., 'Effect of clomiphene on the uterine and oviductal mucosa', *Journal of in Vitro Fertilization and Embryo Transfer* 1, 2, 1984, p. 99.

130 B. Henriet, L. Henriet, D. Hulhove and V. Seynave, 'The Lethal Effect of Superovulation on the embryos', *Abstract, Journal of in Vitro Fertilization and Embryo Transfer* 1, 2, 1984, p. 114.

131 'Danazol May Help Curb Hyperstimulation in Ovulation Induction', *Ob.Gyn.News* 22, 12, 1984, p. 9.

132 P.M. Bolton, 'Bilateral Breast Cancer Associated with Clomiphene', *Lancet*, 3 December 1977, p. 1176.

133 Marian E. Carter and David N. Joyce, 'Ovarian Carcinoma in a Patient Hyperstimulated by Gonadotropin Therapy for In Vitro Fertilization: A Case Report', *Journal of in Vitro Fertilization and Embryo Transfer* 4, 2, 1987, pp. 126-8; Daniel W. Cramer and William R. Welch, 'Determinants of Ovarian Cancer Risk. II. Inferences Regarding Pathogenesis', *Journal of the National Cancer Institute* 71, 4, 1983, pp. 717-21.

134 Personal communication, Professor Eylard Hall, 4 August, 1986.

135 Cunha et al.; Hugh R. Gorwill, Howard D. Steele and Inder R. Sarda, 'Heterotopic Columnar Epithelium and Adenosis in the Vagina of the Mouse After Neonatal Treatment With Clomiphene Citrate', *American Journal of Obstetrics and Gynecology* 144, 5, 1982, pp. 529-32.

136 *Mims Annual* 1984, p. 373.

137 *Mims Annual* 1987, p. 373.

138 *Mims Annual* 1987, p. 373.

139 *Mims Annual* 1987, p. 326.

140 Billy Yee and Joyce Vargyas, 'Multiple follicle development utilising combinations of clomiphene citrate and human menopausal gonadotropins', *Clinical Obstetrics and Gynecology* 29, 1, 1986, pp. 141-7; M.N. Quigley et al., 'Comparison of two clomiphene citrate dosage regimens for follicular recruitment in an in vitro fertilisation program', *Fertility and Sterility* 40, 1983, p. 178; Marrs et al., 'A modified technique of human in vitro fertilisation and embryo transfer', *American Journal of Obstetrics and Gynecology* 147, 1983, p. 318; A. Lopata et al., 'Concepts in human in vitro fertilization and embryo transfer', *Fertility and Sterility* 40, 1983, p. 289.

141 Personal communication from Titia Esser; Klein, *Infertility*.

142 David Healy's letter was widely circulated but not published by the newspapers.

143 Personal communication from Geelong woman.

144 Nick Davidson and Jill Rakusen, *Out of our Hands. What Technology Does to Pregnancy*, Pan Books, London and Sydney, 1982, p. 108.

145 Georgiana Jaciello, 'Chromosome Analysis of Oocytes in Stimulated Cycles', Letters to the Editor, *New England Journal of Medicine* 317, 5, 1987, p. 318.
146 Barbara A. Burton, Contentious Issues of Infertility Therapy—A Consumer's View, Australian Family Planning Annual Conference, March 1985.
147 Klein, *Infertility*.
148 Cited in Laborie.
149 Sandra Blakeslee, 'Trying to Make Money Making "Test-Tube Babies"', *New York Times*, 17 May 1987.
150 J.R. Zorn, P. Boyer, A. Guichard, 'Never on a Sunday: programming for IVF-ET and GIFT', *Lancet*, 14 February 1987, pp. 385-6.
151 Peter Bromwich et al., 'In vitro fertilisation in a small unit in the NHS', *British Medical Journal* 296, 1988, pp. 759-61.
152 Suheil J. Muasher, Jairo E. Garcia, and Howard W. Jones, 'Experience with Diethylstilbestrol-exposed Infertile Women in a Program of in Vitro Fertilisation', *Fertility and Sterility* 42, 1, 1984, pp. 20-4.
153 Ford, p. 39.
154 See Laborie.
155 Laborie; Marcia O'Keefe, 'IVF and Cancer: A Personal Experience', *Issues in Reproduction and Genetic Engineering. Journal of International Feminism Analysis*, 1992, forthcoming.
156 'The cow that sprang from a tube', *New Scientist*, 24 March 1988, p. 27.
157 Calvin Miller, 'When a foetus is a "mother"', *Australian Weekly Doctor*, 27 May 1988.
158 Christine Kilgore, 'Egg donation programs facing ethical issues, donor shortage', and 'New technique boosts prospects of ovum banks', *Ob.Gyn.News* 25, 3, February 1990, pp. 1-16.
159 Charles H. Hendricks, 'Twinning in relation to birth weight, mortality and congenital anomalies', *Obstetrics and Gynecology* 27, 1966, pp. 47-53.
160 John O'Neill, 'For this baby, IVF is no miracle', *Sydney Morning Herald*, 1 January 1988, p. 1.
161 'IVF and GIFT pregnancies...', NPSU, p. 2.
162 Anne L. Rickards et al., 'Extremely low birthweight infants: neurological, psychological, growth and health status beyond five years of age', *Medical Journal of Australia* 147, 16 November 1987, pp. 476-81.
163 Danielle Robinson, 'Bid to save tiny babies questioned by doctors', *Weekend Australian*, 16-17 August 1986.
164 'Rise in multiple births places other babies at risk', *Age*, 17 June 1987, p. 7.
165 Andrew Veitch, 'Odds stacked against multiple babies', *Guardian*, 18 August 1987.
166 Hendricks.
167 'Rise in multiple births...'.

168 Gina Kolata, 'Multiple fetuses raise new issues tied to abortion', *New York Times*, 25 January 1988, p. 15.
169 Dr Birnholz, 'Fetal Reduction aids postgonadotropin multiple pregnancy', *Ob.Gyn.News* 23, 4, 1988; TV interview, *NBC Today Show Live from America*, 3 May 1988.
170 ibid.
171 Ann Treweek, 'One twin terminated, the other survives world-first surgery', *Advertiser*, 9 July 1986, p. 2.
172 Dr Lawrence Platt, quoted in Kolata.
173 A. Demoulin, J.P. Schaaps, R. Bologne and R. Lambotte, 'Is ultrasound monitoring of follicular growth harmless?' *Journal of in Vitro Fertilization and Embryo Transfer* 1, 2, 1984, p. 106.
174 Ruth Hubbard, 'Legal and Policy implications of recent advances in prenatal diagnosis and fetal therapy', *Women's Rights Law Reporter* 7, 3, 1982, p. 208.
175 Philip McIntosh, 'Most medical practice quackery, says doctor', *Age*, 23 September 1986, p. 5.
176 Claire Tedeschi, 'Just how safe is pregnancy scanning?', *Sun-Herald*, 3 February 1985.
177 'At least 75% of maternal deaths considered to be preventable', *Ob.Gyn.News* 21, 9, 1986, p. 14.
178 David Hicks, 'Is sperm dangerous?' *World Medicine*, October 1984, pp. 21–2; Jerome K. Sherman and George W. Jordan, 'Cryosurvival of Chlamydia trachomatis during cryopreservation of human spermatozoa', *Fertility and Sterility* 43, 4, 1985, pp. 664–6.
179 'Four infected by AIDS through donor semen', *Age*, 25 July 1985.
180 Edwin Peterson, Nancy Alexander, Kamran Moghissi, 'A.I.D. and AIDS —too close for comfort', *Fertility and Sterility* 49, 2, 1988, pp. 209–11.
181 Klein, *Infertility*; dos Reis; Gena Corea, personal communication on the Zenaide Project; analysis to be published in 1992 by The Institute on Women and Technology, MIT, Massachusetts.
182 Ann Treweek, 'Coroner investigates IVF patient deaths', *Australian Doctor Weekly*, 5 May 1988; see also Gena Corea 'Surrogacy: Making the Links', in Klein, *Infertility*; *Age*, 29 November 1988 cited in *FINRRAGE newsletter*, March 1989, p. 5.
183 Heather Waby, "The tragic side of the IVF program', *Woman's Day*, 28 March 1988, pp. 12–13; Jane Phillips, Jeff Jenkins, 'Shot mum's tragic secret', *Sun*, 17 February 1988.
184 R. Anderson, 'IVF failures need counselling', *Age*, 24 February 1988.
185 Christine Crowe, 'Women want it': in-vitro fertilization and women's motivations for participation', *Women's Studies International Forum* 8, 6, 1985, pp. 547–52; Barbara Burton, Contentious issues of infertility therapy—a consumer's view, paper presented to the Annual meeting of the Australian Family Planning Association, Lorne, March 1985; Klein, *Exploitation* and *Infertility*.

186 Crowe, p. 550.
187 Burton, p. 5.
188 Crowe.
189 Klein, *Exploitation*, p. 19.
190 Burton, p. 9.
191 Personal communication, 25 June 1985.
192 These quotations from R. Klein, *Exploitation*, pp. 20, 27.
193 Burton, p. 6.
194 Burton, pp. 8, 7.
195 Klein, *Exploitation*, p. 30.
196 ibid., p. 33.
197 Klein, *Exploitation*, p. 34.
198 ibid., pp. 34–5.
199 Burton, p. 12.
200 Klein, *Exploitation*, p. 40.
201 Diagnosis Pty Ltd, Table 8.
202 Lasker and Borg, p. 30.
203 Klein, *Exploitation*, p. 36.
204 'Consultation on the place of in vitro fertilization in infertility care', World Health Organization, Regional Office for Europe, Copenhagen, 18–22 June 1990.

2. THE MASCULINE DREAM OF QUALITY CONTROL: GENETIC ENGINEERING

1 Viola Roggencamp, 'Abortion of a special kind', in Rita Arditti, Renate Duelli Klein and Shelley Minden (eds), *Test Tube Women: What Future For Motherhood?*, Pandora Press, London, 1984, pp. 273–4.
2 Roberta Steinbacher, 'Futuristic implications of sex preselection', in *The Custom-Made Child?—Women-Centred Perspectives*, Humana Press, New Jersey, 1981; Janice Raymond, *Man-Made Women: How New Reproductive Technologies Affect Women*, Hutchison, London, 1985, p. 11; Gena Corea, *The Mother Machine: Reproductive Technologies from Artificial Insemination to Artificial Wombs*, Harper & Row, New York, 1985, p. 188. Mary Anne Warren has also given it the misleading term 'gendercide', assuming what she calls 'gender-neutral' language (Mary Anne Warren. *Gendercide: The Implications of Sex Selection*, Rowman & Allanheld, New Jersey, 1985); yet the term is misleading, because history shows periods of systematic elimination of women purely because of their sex as in the practice of female infanticide, in the witch-hunts, and suttee (wife-burning), which do not have analogies in male history.
3 Bob Johnstone, 'Japanese choose their baby's sex', *New Scientist* 110, 1513, 1986, p. 22.

4 'Infant sex pre-selection controversy aids marketeers', *Health Care Marketing Report*, November 1986, p. 7; Vibhuti Patel, Amniocentesis —an abuse of advanced scientific technique, Paper presented at XIth World Congress of Sociology, New Delhi, 18–22 August 1986, p. 9.
5 Jonathan Hewitt, 'Preconceptional sex selection', *British Journal of Hospital Medicine* 37, 2, 1987, p. 151.
6 Ursula Mittwoch, 'The race to be male', *New Scientist*, 22 October 1988, p. 38.
7 Lynda Birke, 'Genetic clues to the development of sex', *New Scientist*, 17 December 1988, p. 14; Christopher Joyce, 'Geneticists find the gene that determines sex', *New Scientist*, 24–31 December 1987, p. 29.
8 'Sex predetermined in test-tube birth', *Boston Globe*, 6 August 1986; Gena Corea, 'Surrogacy: Making the Links', in Renate Klein (ed.), *Infertility: Women Speak Out About Their Experiences of Reproductive Medicine*, Pandora Press, London, 1989, p. 135.
9 John D. West, John R. Gosden, Roslyn R. Angell, Nicholas D. Hastie, Samuel S. Thatcher, Anna F. Glasier, David T. Baird, 'Sexing the human pre-embryo by DNA-DNA in situ hybridization', *Lancet*, 13 June 1987, p. 1345.
10 Kathy Johnston, 'Sex of embryos known', *Nature* 327, 1987, p. 547.
11 Alan Handyside, 'Sex and the single cell', *New Scientist*, 21 April 1990, pp. 18–19.
12 Radhakrishna Rao, 'Move to stop sex-test abortion', *Nature* 324, 1986, p. 202; Radhakrishna Rao, 'Move to ban sex determination', *Nature* 331, 1986, p. 467.
13 Bharati Sadasivam, 'The silent scream', *Illustrated Weekly of India*, 14 September 1986, p. 39.
14 Vibhuti Patel, Amniocentesis—abuse of advanced scientific technique, paper presented at the XIth World Congress of Sociology, New Delhi, 18–22 August 1986, p. 1.
15 Cited in Sadasivam, p. 40.
16 Sadasivam.
17 Bill Mellor, 'Predetermining sex threat to Australian male–female ratio', *Sun-Herald*, 13 December 1987, p. 58.
18 Maj Hulten, Paul Needham, Jessie L. Watt and Mike Griffiths, 'Preventing feticide', *Nature* 325, 1987, p. 190.
19 'Infant sex pre-selection controversy aids marketeers', *Healthcare Marketing Report*, November 1986, p. 7; 'Potential impact of increase in sex pre-selection', *Ob.Gyn.News* 25, 6, 1990, p. 39.
20 Mellor.
21 Anne Woodman, 'Tests "led to abortions" ', *Sun*, 23 October 1987.
22 Nancy Williamson, *Sons or Daughters: A Cross Cultural Survey of Parental Preferences*, Sage, London, 1976.

23 Hilary Rose, 'Victorian values in the test-tube: the politics of reproductive science and technology', in Michelle Stanworth (ed.), *Reproductive Technologies: Gender, Motherhood and Medicine*, Polity Press, Cambridge, 1987, p. 169.
24 Steinbacher.
25 'Survey shows most don't want to select infant's sex', *Ob.Gyn.News* 22, 2, 1987.
26 John Postgate, 'Bat's chance in hell', *New Scientist* 5, 1973, pp. 11-16.
27 M. Guttenberg and P. Secord, *Too Many Women? The Sex Ratio Question*, Sage, London, 1983, p. 2.
28 Colin Campbell, 'The manchild pill', *Psychology Today*, August 1976, p. 88.
29 Barbara Katz Rothman, *The Tentative Pregnancy*, Penguin, New York, 1986, p. 150.
30 Don Kirk, 'Europe fumbles toward agreement on embryo research', *New Scientist*, 19 November 1988, p. 20.
31 Sian Griffiths, 'Big rise in embryo research', *Age*, 13 May 1988. For the ongoing debate on embryo experimentation in Australia, see, for example, Michael Pirrie, 'All clear for research on 80 embryos', *Age*, 14 July 1988, p. 1; Jackie Allender, 'Vic go-ahead for embryo experiments', *Australian*, 15 July 1988, p. 4; Michael Pirrie, 'New IVF research method prompts a debate on ethics', *Age*, 15 July 1988; Christine Ewing, 'The case against embryo experimentation: a feminist perspective', *Legal Service Bulletin* 14, 3, 1989, pp. 109-12.
32 Griffiths.
33 Results from a questionnaire carried out by a group called Concern for the Infertile Couple—A Survey of Infertile Couples' Attitudes Towards IVF in Western Australia—December 1984, p. 9.
34 Helen Bequaert Holmes and Tjeerd Tynstra, 'In vitro fertilisation in The Netherlands: experiences and opinions of Dutch women', *Journal of In Vitro Fertilization and Embryo Transfer* 4, 2, 1987, pp. 116-23.
35 Select Committee on the Human Embryo Experimentation Bill 1985, Commonwealth of Australia, *Hansard*, 24 April 1986, p. 1758.
36 Andrew Veitch, '"Let embryos grow in pigs" plea', *Guardian*, 19 December 1984; John Illman, 'Test tube baby team seek animal implants', *London Daily Mail*, 19 December 1984; David Fletcher, 'Embryos in animals planned', *Daily Telegraph*, 19 December 1984.
37 Johanna Riegler and Aurelia Weikert, 'Product egg: egg selling in an Austrian IVF clinic', *Reproductive and Genetic Engineering: Journal of International Feminist Analysis* 1, 3, 1988, p. 222.
38 Jane Southward, 'IVF use of egg donors raises legal problems', *Sun-Herald*, 11 February 1990; Michael Pirrie, 'Hospital seeks egg donors', *Age*, 27 October 1989.

39 Jackie Allender, 'Embryo tests to detect genetic ills', *Australian*, 27 December 1989, pp. 1, 2.

40 *IVF and GIFT pregnancies Australia and New Zealand 1988*, National Perinatal Statistics Unit, Sydney, 1990.

41 Mike Rayner, 'Experiments on embryos: stick to the facts', *New Scientist*, 27 February 1986, p. 54.

42 Jane Ford, 'Sheep will grow woollier on a bioengineered diet', *New Scientist*, 10 March 1988, p. 24.

43 Peter Quiddington, 'Genetic breakthrough could mean dotty daisies', *Australian*, 13 December 1988.

44 Ben Bremner, 'Organisms to order herald a revolution in biotechnology', *Australian*, 1 November 1988, p. 50; Jane Ford, 'This little pig rushed to market', *New Scientist*, 28 April 1988, p. 27; Jane Ford, 'Sheep will grow', p. 24; Graeme O'Neill, 'Gene maps for a slimmer chicken', *Age*, 6 June 1988; Jane Ford, 'Gene transplant yields "super sheep"', *Australian*, 25 June 1986, p. 11.

45 Bob Beale, 'Scientists create the test-tube "brahford"', *Sydney Morning Herald*, 28 November 1987.

46 Simon Hadlington, 'Transgenic sow', *Nature*, 2 July 1987.

47 Graeme O'Neill, 'Scientists want cows to become gene harvesters', *Age*, 16 July 1987, p. 3.

48 Ian Anderson, 'A mouse with a human immune system', *New Scientist*, 14 January 1989, pp. 33–4.

49 Views, *British Medical Journal* 297, 6 August 1988, p. 432.

50 Christopher Joyce, 'Patent on mouse breaks new ground', *New Scientist*, 21 April 1988, p. 23.

51 Ford, 'This little pig'; Carol Ezzell, 'First ever animal patent issued in United States', *Nature* 332, 1988, p. 668.

52 Ford, 'This little pig', p. 27.

53 Joyce, 21 April 1988, p. 23.

54 Rhonda Dredge, 'Case of the super pig that went to market', *Age*, 2 May 1990, p. 13; Graeme O'Neill, 'The issue is the right to know', *Age*, 2 May 1990, p. 13.

55 Barbara Ford, 'Parent of the apes', *Omni*, November 1981, p. 39.

56 Daniel Golden, 'Playing God?', *Boston Globe*, 3 May 1987.

57 ibid., p. A23.

58 DNA (deoxyribonucleic acid) is the molecule of heredity. Most of the DNA is organised into chromosomes inside cells. Each cell of the body has 46 chromosomes, except eggs and sperm which contain 23 each. A chromosome is made up of two strands of DNA which twist around each other in a shape known as the double helix. DNA is a long macromolecule. Each strand of DNA is made up of smaller molecules called nucleotides. These nucleotides occur in a defined sequence and can only pair with particular nucleotides on the second strand of DNA to create the twist which is the double helix. This is called base-pairing.

A gene is a piece of DNA within a chromosome that is said to have a specific function or which may be multifunctional. Genes determine the kinds of proteins (e.g. antibodies, hormones, enzymes) that are made by cells and which maintain individual cells and the whole organism. Genes carry the instructions for making specific cell products and many of these are identifiable; for instance, we do know the genes which manufacture antibodies. But in human cells there are 50 000 to 100 000 genes, which makes it difficult to locate the tasks of all individual genes, especially when more than one gene may contribute to a function. Also, some of the DNA has no apparent function. The theory is that genes are not operating or 'switched on' all the time, only when necessary. For example, scientists are trying to determine why a gene will inappropriately switch on to create rapidly developing cancer cells.

A marker gene may be a seemingly harmless DNA variation that occurs in people who have a genetic illness for which the gene is as yet unknown. The marker gene is said to be in the vicinity of the problem gene.

59 Sharon Kingman, 'Buried treasure in human genes', *New Scientist*, 8 July 1989, pp. 12–13; Christopher Joyce, 'US faces demands for secrecy on genome programme', *New Scientist*, 18 November 1989, p. 5; 'The race for the human genome', *British Medical Journal* 297, 1988, p. 577; Carol Ezzell, 'Another report smiles on human genome sequencing project', *Nature* 332, 1988, p. 769.

60 'Gene causing cystic fibrosis may soon be found', *Ob.Gyn.News* 23, 15, August 1988.

61 'Genetic defects found earlier', *Herald*, 20 July 1988.

62 'Fetal diagnosis of thalassemia by DNA analysis 95% accurate', *Ob.Gyn.News* 22, 1, 1987.

63 Georgina Ferry, 'No extra genes in Alzheimer's disease', *New Scientist*, 19 November 1987, p. 32.

64 'Isolated sect provides clues for genetic study', *Australian*, 5 July 1987.

65 Christine Ewing, 'Tailored genes: IVF, genetic engineering and eugenics', *Reproductive and Genetic Engineering. Journal of International Feminist Analysis* 1, 1, 1988, pp. 31–40. Ewing has argued that manic depression suffers from subjectiveness in diagnosis because the symptoms are largely behavioural. As with many of these studies, researchers attempt to exclude environmental factors by looking at specific and isolated communities. But not everyone in susceptible families develops these conditions.

66 'Genes identified that might cause one-third of manic depression', *Ob.Gyn.News* 22, 11, 1987, p. 22.

67 Gail Vines, 'Lung cancer genes located', *New Scientist*, 17 December 1987, p. 12.

68 Christopher Joyce, 'Americans plan gene therapy on people', *New Scientist*, 4 August 1988, p. 24; 'Pioneering therapy with genes moves a stage closer', *New Scientist*, 15 October 1988, p. 27; Christopher Joyce, 'US approves trials with gene therapy', *New Scientist*, 11 August 1990, p. 7.

69 Susan Downie, 'Early detection to avoid diabetes', *Herald*, 15 March 1988, p. 9.

70 *Australian Women's Weekly*, January 1988.

71 Ricki Lewis, 'Genetic-marker testing: are we ready for it?', *Issues in Science and Technology*, Fall 1989, pp. 76–82.

72 ibid.

73 David M. Danks, 'Progress towards gene therapy', *Nature* 333, 1988, p. 202.

74 Glennys Bell, 'Designer genes', *Bulletin*, 7 February 1989.

75 *Genetic Manipulation*, Discussion Paper No. 11, Law Reform Commission of Victoria, 1988, p. 15.

76 Paula Bradish, 'From genetic counselling and genetic analysis, to genetic ideal and genetic fate?', in Patricia Spallone and Deborah Lynn Steinberg (eds), *Made To Order: The Myth of Reproductive and Genetic Progress*, Pergamon Press, Oxford, 1987, p. 99.

77 Golden, p. A21.

78 Christopher Joyce, 'Americans confident about biotechnology', *New Scientist*, 21 July 1988, p. 25.

79 Richard Saltus, 'Biotech firms compete in genetic diagnosis', *Science* 234, 1986, p. 1319.

80 loc. cit.

81 Jane McLoughlin, 'Playing Russian roulette with employees', *Guardian*, 10 July 1986.

82 Harold Schmeck, 'Crystal ball is ethically dark', *Age*, 3 November 1986.

83 Robyn Williams, *The Science Show*, ABC Radio, 4 February 1989.

84 *Genetic Manipulation*, 1988, p. 14.

85 Susan Wright, 'Genetic engineering: the risks are real', *Christianity and Crisis* 43, 19 September 1983, p. 332; Myles Harris, 'Splitting the gene, not the atom', *Age*, 11 October 1987, p. 5; 'DNA and defence', *New Scientist*, 17 December 1988, p. 7.

86 Anne McLaren, 'Can we diagnose genetic disease in pre-embryos?', *New Scientist*, 10 December 1987, p. 42.

87 Glennys Bell, 'Genes that don't fit', *Bulletin*, 5 January 1988.

88 Alison Davis, 'Ethical issues in prenatal diagnosis', *British Medical Journal* 288, 1984, p. 1977; personal communication from Alison Davis, 5 October 1985.

89 Marsha Saxton, 'Prenatal screening and discriminatory attitudes about disability', in Elaine Hoffmann Baruch, Amadeo F. D'Adamo and Joni Seager (eds), *Embryos, Ethics, and Women's Rights: Exploring the New Reproductive Technology*, The Haworth Press, New York, 1988, p. 218.

90 ibid., p. 224.
91 Sally Hughes, 'A good test but where can you take it?', *Guardian*, 7 July 1986.
92 Christopher Nolan, *Under The Eye of The Clock*, Pan, London, 1987.
93 Katz Rothman, p. 238.
94 Ruth Hubbard, 'Eugenics: new tools, old ideas', in Baruch, D'Adama and Seager (eds).
95 Gail Vines, 'Test-tube pioneer fears rise of eugenics', *New Scientist*, 9 October 1986, p. 17.
96 Ewing, Hubbard; Hugh Trevor-Roper, 'Seas of unreason', *Nature* 313, 1985, p. 407.
97 Hubbard, p. 228.
98 Kay Daniels and Mary Murnane, *Uphill All The Way: A Documentary History of Women in Australia*, University of Queensland Press, Brisbane, 1980, pp. 129, 130, 135, 144.
99 Robert J. Lifton, *The Nazi Doctors*, Macmillan, London, 1987, pp. 16, xii.
100 Trevor-Roper, p. 407; Heidrun Kaupen-Haas, 'Experimental obstetrics and national socialism: the conceptual basis of reproductive technology today', *Reproductive and Genetic Engineering. Journal of International Feminist Analysis* 1, 2, 1988, pp. 127–32.
101 Myles Harris, 'Splitting the gene not the atom', *Age*, 11 October 1987, p. 5.
102 Cited in Michelle Stanworth, 'The deconstruction of motherhood', in Stanworth (ed.), *Reproductive Technologies: Gender, Motherhood and Medicine*, Polity Press, Cambridge, 1987, p. 30.
103 Cited in Jocelynne Scutt, 'Women's bodies, patriarchal principles', in Jocelynne Scutt (ed.), *The Baby Machine*, McCulloch Publishing, Melbourne, 1988, p. 218.
104 Stanworth, p. 31.
105 Hubbard, p. 232.
106 Peter Wheale and Ruth McNally. *Genetic Engineering: Catastrophe or Utopia?* Harvester, Wheatsheaf, Hemel Hempstead, Herts, 1988, p. 274.

3. WOMAN AS A DISSOLVING CAPSULE: THE CHALLENGE OF FETAL PERSONHOOD

1 Advertisement, *Ob.Gyn.News*, August 1988.
2 'Fiberscope permits direct visualization of the fetus during labour', *Ob.Gyn.News* 22, 2, 1987, p. 1.
3 Michael Harrison, 'Unborn: historical perspective of the fetus as a patient', *Pharos*, 1982, p. 19.
4 ibid., p. 22. Marilyn Frye argues that men are parasitical in their relationships with women and therefore identify with the fetus, which also feeds off the woman. Many men therefore try to restrict

abortion because they feel that women who can cut one lifeline can cut theirs too. 'In the eyes of the other parasite, the image of the wholly self-determined abortion, involving not even a ritual submission to male veto power, is the mirror image of death.' See 'Some reflections on separation and power', *The Politics of Reality: essays in feminist theory*, Crossing Press, New York, 1983, p. 101.

5 Harrison, p. 24.

6 P.M. Sharples, P.L. Hope and A.R. Wilkinson, 'False positive in prenatal diagnosis of cystic fibrosis', *Lancet*, 12 March 1988, p. 595.

7 Caroline Whitebeck, 'Fetal imaging and fetal monitoring: finding the ethical issues', in Baruch, D'Adamo and Seager (eds), *Embryos, Ethics and Women's Rights: Exploring The New Reproductive Technologies*, The Haworth Press, New York, 1988, p. 51. See also Jeff Cogen, 'Obs. still using EFM despite lack of efficacy data', *Ob.Gyn.News* 25, 11, 1990.

8 R.E. Myers, 'Maternal anxiety and fetal death,' in L. Zichella and P. Pancheri (eds), *Psychoendocrinology in Reproduction*, North Holland Biomedical Press, Elsevier, Holland, 1979; Nancy K. Rhoden, 'The judge in the delivery room: the emergence of court-ordered caesareans', *California Law Review* 74, 6, 1986, p. 2016.

9 Rhoden, p. 2017.

10 Ruth Hubbard, 'Legal and policy implications of recent advances in prenatal diagnosis and fetal therapy', *Women's Rights Law Reporter* 7, 3, 1982, p. 202.

11 Frank Chervenak and Lawrence McCullough, 'Perinatal ethics: a practical method of analysis of obligations to mother and fetus', *Obstetrics and Gynecology* 66, 3, 1985, pp. 442–6.

12 Sherman E. Elias and George J. Annas, 'Perspectives on Fetal surgery', *American Journal of Obstetrics and Gynecology*, 145, 7, 1983, p. 810.

13 Hubbard.

14 Hubbard; John C. Fletcher, 'Healing before birth: an ethical dilemma', *Technology Review*, January 1984, p. 34.

15 Watson Bowes and Brad Selgestad, 'Fetal versus maternal rights: medical and legal perspectives', *Obstetrics and Gynecology* 58, 2, 1981, p. 211.

16 Louise Chunn, 'Foetal rights: more than a mother can bear?', *Elle*, July 1988, pp. 33–4.

17 'Drama in the womb: a matter of life and death winds up in court', *Los Angeles Times*, 25 December 1987.

18 Janet Gallagher, 'The fetus and the law: whose life is it anyway?', *Ms*, September 1984, p. 62.

19 Dana Rubin, 'Mother accused of harming her fetus', *San Jose Mercury News*, 2 October 1986, p. 1.

20 ibid., p. 1.

21 Joanne Jacobs, 'Protecting the fetus at women's expense: the slippery slope of the fetal abuse case', *San Jose Mercury News*, 6 October 1986.
22 Sally Koch, 'Treatment of gravida against her wishes debated', *Ob.Gyn.News* 20, 9, 1985, pp. 1, 20.
23 Veronika E.B. Kolder, Janet Gallagher and Michael T. Parsons, Court ordered obstetrical interventions, *New England Journal of Medicine* 316, 1987, p. 1192.
24 'Urges strict criteria for forced intervention on behalf of fetus', *Ob.Gyn.News* 23, 2, 1988, pp. 3, 31.
25 Sarah Ahmann, 'ACOG opposes court-ordered treatment of pregnant women', *Ob.Gyn.News* 22, 18, 1987, pp. 1, 19.
26 'Child abuse begins before birth: doctor', *Adelaide Advertiser*, 13 July 1986, p. 1.
27 Christine Overall, *Ethics in Human Reproduction. A Feminist Analysis*, Allen & Unwin, Boston, 1987, p. 3.
28 Cited in Hubbard, p. 215.
29 Janine Perrett, 'Mother or foetus: who has the right?' *Australian*, 5 August 1988.
30 'Foetal seizure unlawful, says Canadian court', *Age*, 11 August 1988.
31 'Evaluating job stress, risk for pregnant patient', *Ob.Gyn.News* 22, 11, 1987, p. 3.
32 Rosalind Pollack Petchesky, *Abortion and Woman's Choice: The State, Sexuality and Reproductive Freedom*, Longman, New York, 1984, p. 350; Thomas H. Murray, 'Who do fetal protection policies really protect?', *Technology Review*, October 1985, pp. 12–13, 20.
33 Cited in Petchesky (her emphasis), p. 351.
34 Frank Swoboda, 'High court will be asked to review company's "fetal protection policy"', *Washington Post*, 7 January 1990, p. 4.
35 Petchesky, p. 352; Rayna Rapp, 'Moral pioneers: women, men and fetuses on a frontier of reproductive technology', in Baruch, D'Adamo and Seager, p. 102.
36 Hubbard.
37 Rapp.
38 Barbara Katz Rothman, *The Tentative Pregnancy; Prenatal Diagnosis and the Future of Motherhood*, Penguin, New York, 1986, pp. 114–15.
39 'Say amniocentesis raises risk of fetal loss, infant respiratory ills', *Ob.Gyn.News* 21, 19, 1986, p. 39.
40 'Abortion risk up with age in chorionic villi sampling', *Ob.Gyn.News* 23, 4, 1988.
41 *British Medical Journal*, 1977, p. 1237.
42 Judith A. Bell, John H. Pearn and Arabella Smith, 'Prenatal cyrogenetic diagnosis. Amniotic cell culture versus chorion villus sampling', *Medical Journal of Australia* 146, 1987, p. 28.

43 Jeffrey E. Green, Andrew Dorfmann, Shirley Jones, Samuel Bender, Laurel Patton and Joseph Schulman, 'Chorionic villus sampling: experience with an initial 940 cases', *Obstetrics and Gynecology* 71, 2, 1988, p. 208.
44 'Urges study of long-term effects of chorionic test' and 'Chorionic villus sampling accuracy, safety debated', *Ob.Gyn.News* 21, 9, 1986, p. 23.
45 'Ultrasound guides surgeon's scalpel', *Age*, 19 July 1985, p. 3.
46 'New invasive ob. procedures assessed; some still require work', *Ob.Gyn.News* 21, 21, 1986, p. 27.
47 Calvin Miller, 'Surgery on foetus corrects defects', *Herald*, 24 August 1988, p. 2.
48 Miriam Tucker, 'Fetal surgery viewed with "cautious optimism"', *Ob.Gyn.News* 21, 20, 1986, p. 44.
49 Elias and Annas, pp. 808, 810.
50 Ian Anderson, 'Fetal operation opens up legal controversy', *New Scientist*, 16 October 1986, p. 20.
51 Robin Marantz Henig, 'Saving babies before birth', *New York Times*, 28 February 1982, pp. 46, 48.
52 Hubbard, p. 209.
53 'Recommend halt to most in vitro shunt procedures for fetal hydrocephalus', *Ob.Gyn.News* 21, 9, 1986, p. 36.
54 Hubbard, p. 210.
55 'Advances in fetal surgery "self-limiting"', *Ob.Gyn.News* 22, 2, 1987, p. 46.
56 Miller.
57 Calvin Miller, 'When a foetus is a mother', *Australian Doctor Weekly*, 27 May 1988.
58 Gail Vines, 'Transplanted eggs can create ovaries', *New Scientist*, 10 February 1990, p. 12.
59 Ian Anderson, 'Brain graft revives sufferers from Parkinson's disease', *New Scientist*, 14 January 1988, p. 28; Jeff Hecht, 'Brain implant treats Huntington's disease', *New Scientist*, 21 April 1988, p. 22; Philip McIntosh, 'Call for guidelines on foetal tissue', *Age*, 27 July 1985; Georgina Ferry, 'New cells for old brains', *New Scientist*, 24 March 1988, pp. 45–58; Susan Downie, *Baby Making: The Technology and Ethics*, The Bodley Head, London, 1988.
60 Ferry, p. 58.
61 'Fetuses and Parkinsonism', *Nature* 332, 1988, p. 667.
62 Ferry, p. 57.
63 Neville Hodgkinson, 'Brain tissue transplants inflame ethical and emotional furore', *Australian*, 20 April 1988.
64 Mary B. Mahowald, Jenny Silver and Robert A. Ratcheson, 'The ethical operations in transplanting fetal tissue', *Hastings Center Report*, February 1987, pp. 9–15.
65 McIntosh.
66 Susanna Rodell, 'The brain cell dilemma', *Herald*, 4 May 1988.

67 Ferry, p. 57.
68 Hodgkinson.
69 Christopher Hanson, 'Baby farming: the modern moral dilemma', *Australian*, 26 November 1987.
70 Tania Ewing, 'The bioethics of foetal brain transplants', *Medical Observer*, 27 May 1988, p. 5; Dan McDonnell, 'Saviour is born; sceptics uneasy', *Sunday Herald*, 8 April 1990; Maree Curtis, 'A baby to save my boy', *Sun*, 7 April 1990, pp. 1, 2.
71 'Foetuses sold to labs, BBC says', *Sydney Morning Herald*, 1 November 1988.
72 Susanna Rodell, 'Aborted foetuses cleared for brain transplants', *Herald*, 11 May 1988.
73 Jonathan Adams, 'Federal panel terms fetal tissue research ethically acceptable', *Ob.Gyn.News* 23, 20, 1988, p. 1.
74 Christopher Reed, 'Campaign against foetal experiments', *Age*, 10 March 1988.
75 Sally McMillan, 'When a mother's grief over a dying son gives rise to joy', *Australian*, 18 December 1987; David Ferrell, 'Babies, or organ quarries', *Age*, 20 November 1987.
76 Anne Scheck, 'Effort to harvest anencephalics' organs suspended', *Ob.Gyn.News* 23, 21, 1988, pp. 2, 13.
77 Calvin Miller, 'Babies, transplants—and ethics', *Herald*, 19 October 1988.
78 Michael Harrison, 'Organ procurement for children: the anencephalic fetus as donor', *Lancet*, 13 December 1986, p. 1384.
79 '... as European Ministers outlaw trade in human organs', *New Scientist*, 10 December 1987, p. 16.
80 Janice Raymond, 'Children for organ export?', *Reproductive and Genetic Engineering: Journal of International Feminist Analysis* 2, 3, 1989, p. 237, p. 244. See also 'Babies were to be killed for their organs', *Herald*, 8 July 1988.
81 Dena Kleiman, 'When abortion becomes birth: a dilemma of medical ethics shaken by new advances', *New York Times*, 15 February 1984, p. B1.
82 Daniel Farber, 'Abortion economics', *The New Republic*, 14–21 July 1986, p. 15.
83 ibid., p. 15.
84 Rapp, p. 113.
85 Hubbard, p. 218.

4. THE DEPERSONALISATION OF BIRTH MOTHERS: SO-CALLED 'SURROGACY'

1 Elizabeth Kane, *Birth Mother*, Harcourt Brace Jovanovich, San Diego, 1988, p. 277.
2 Cynthia Gorney, 'For love and money', *California Magazine*, October 1983.

3 Nancy Barrass, 'Women who experienced surrogacy speak out', in Renate Klein (ed.), *Infertility: Women Speak Out About Their Experiences of Reproductive Medicine*, Pandora Press, London, 1989, p. 156.
4 Susan Ince, 'Inside the surrogate industry', in Rita Arditti, Renate Duelli Klein and Shelley Minden (eds), *Test-Tube Women. What Future For Motherhood*, Pandora Press, London, 1984.
5 See Klein
6 Rita Arditti, 'A summary of some recent developments on surrogacy in the United States', *Reproductive and Genetic Engineering, Journal of International Feminist Analysis* 1, 1, 1988, p. 52.
7 Cited in Arditti, pp. 54, 56.
8 Barrass, p. 157.
9 Gorney, p. 96.
10 Colin Dale, 'Surrogates', *Sunday Press*, 3 June 1984, p. 22.
11 Alejandra Munoz, 'Women who experienced surrogacy speak out', in Klein.
12 Nicholas Timmins, 'Why I am having a baby for my sister', *Times*, 23 November 1984, pp. 10-11.
13 Susan Peak and Lyn Cossar, 'Epworth ethics board refused surrogacy case', *Herald*, 13 April 1988; Peter Terry, 'IVF babies "created against ethical advice" ', *Herald*, 21 October 1988, p. 1; Rosemary West, 'Victoria's first IVF surrogate mother may also be the last', *Age*, 20 April 1988.
14 Elizabeth Kane, *Birth Mother*, Macmillan, Melbourne, 1990, p. 280, (Epilogue).
15 John Leeton in John Monks, ' "I'll have your surrogate baby": Twins' amazing pact', *New Idea*, 15 September 1989, pp. 12-13; Response by members of the Monash University Bioethics Centre titled 'Comments on the Report on the disposition of embryos produced in *in vitro* fertilisation', to the Social Responsibilities Commission of the Anglican General Synod, 18 February 1985.
16 'Daughter has mother's baby', *Australian*, 24 October 1988; Susan Jimison, 'Girl gives birth to her own brother', *Weekly World News*, 6 December 1988, p. 15.
17 Suzanne Brenner, 'Granny and the triplets come home', *Woman's Day*, 11 January 1988, pp. 2-3; Peter Younghusband, 'Delivery day for surrogate gran', *Australian*, 24 September 1987; Chris Erasmus, 'Mother gives birth to daughter's babies', *Age*, 2 October 1987; M.C. Michelow, J. Bernstein, M.J. Jacobson, J.L. McLoughlin, D. Rubenstein, A.I. Hacking, S. Preddy, and I.J. van der Wat, 'Mother-daughters in *in vitro* fertilization triplet pregnancy', *Journal of in Vitro Fertilization and Embryo Transfer* 5, 1988, pp. 31-4.
18 Deborah Stone, 'The case of the IVF grandmother', *Sunday Age*, 30 December 1990, p. 9.

19 Philip J. Parker, The Psychology of the pregnant surrogate mother: a newly updated report of a longitudinal study, revised and presented in part to the American Orthopsychiatric Association Meeting, Toronto, 9 April 1984.
20 Gena Corea, *The Mother Machine*, Harper & Row, New York, 1985, p. 229.
21 Aileen Berry, 'Our morals puzzle surrogates' go between', *Age*, 1 August 1984; Trudi McIntosh, 'American here to sell surrogate dreams', *Australian*, 1 August 1984.
22 Annette Gartland, 'This woman will rent you a womb...for £15,000', *Irish Times*, 25 May 1984.
23 Corea.
24 R. Miller, 'Surrogate parenting: an infant industry presents society with legal, ethical questions', *Ob.Gyn.News* 18, 3, 1983.
25 Alan Rassaby, 'Surrogate motherhood: the position and problems of substitutes', in William Walters and Peter Singer (eds), *Test-Tube Babies. A Guide to Moral Questions, Present Techniques and Future Possibilities*, Oxford University Press, Melbourne, 1982, p. 102.
26 Lucy Twomey, 'Surrogate motherhood: a blessing or exploitation?', *Australian*, 2 May 1983.
27 Ute Winkler, 'New US know-how in Frankfurt—a "surrogate mother" agency', *Reproductive and Genetic Engineering. Journal of International Feminist Analysis* 1, 2, 1988, pp. 205-7.
28. Judith N. Lasker and Susan Borg, *In Search of Parenthood: Coping With Infertility and Hi-Tech Conception*, Beacon Press, Boston, 1987.
29 Klein.
30 Sue Morgan, 'Legislation on surrogate motherhood "out of date", says US lawyer', *Sydney Morning Herald*, 2 August 1984.
31 Tricia Harper, 'Surrogate motherhood: should we follow this US example?', *Institute of Family Studies Newsletter* 12, 1985, p. 12.
32 Gorney, p. 153.
33 Lasker and Borg, p. 77.
34 Diana Brahams, 'Surrogacy, adoption and custody', *Lancet*, 4 April 1987, p. 817.
35 David Fletcher, 'Surrogate mothers take on the law', *Sydney Morning Herald*, 18 June 1986.
36 Corea, p. 245.
37 Stephen Lynas, 'Moment when I left baby Cotton', *Daily Mail*, 16 January 1985, p. 5.
38 Gorney, p. 95.
39 Mary Daly, *Gyn/Ecology: The Metaethics of Radical Feminism*, Beacon Press, Boston, 1978, pp. 374-5.
40 Lou Benson, *Images, Heroes and Self-Perceptions: The Struggle For Identity—From Mask-Wearing to Authenticity*, Prentice-Hall, New Jersey, 1974, p. 53.

41 Andrea Dworkin, *Right Wing Women: The Politics of Domesticated Females*, The Women's Press, London, 1978, p. 21.
42 William James, 'The self', in Chad Gordon and Kenneth J. Gergen (eds), *The Self In Social Interaction*, vol. 1: *Classic and contemporary Perspectives*, Wiley, New York, 1968, p. 42.
43 David Gelman and Daniel Shapiro, 'Infertility: babies by contract', *Newsweek*, 4 November 1985, pp. 74–7; 'Other mothers: the surrogate debate', *Public Welfare*, Fall 1983, p. 12.
44 John Grossman, 'Why I was a surrogate mother', *Sun-Herald*, 18 August 1985.
45 Jacky Hyams, 'The surrogate mum who couldn't give up her son', *Australian Women's Weekly*, June 1988, p. 11.
46 Emma Dally, 'The story of a surrogate mother', *Observer*, 13 January 1985, p. 9.
47 Foster, in Klein, p. 150.
48 Lasker and Borg, p. 117.
49 Kane, in Klein, p. 160.
50 Sue Reid, 'Amazing mum gives birth to her own grandchildren', *New Idea*, 26 October 1987, p. 6.
51 Corea.
52 Dava Sobel, 'Surrogate mothers: why women volunteer', *New York Times*, 29 June 1981, p.B5; Philip J. Parker, 'Motivation of surrogate mothers: initial findings', *American Journal of Psychiatry* 140, 1983, pp. 117–18.
53 Mary Beth Whitehead, 'Women who experienced surrogacy speak out', in Klein p. 140; Barrass, in Klein, pp. 154–5.
54 Lasker and Borg, pp. 84, 82, 85.
55 Gorney, p. 150.
56 Lasker and Borg, p. 79.
57 Polly Toynbee, 'Bye, baby Cotton, for love and money', *Sydney Morning Herald*, 13 July 1985, p. 43.
58 Dally.
59 Bob Cameron, 'The search for a surrogate mother', *New Idea*, 12 April 1986, p. 9.
60 Martin Daly, 'Mothers the law rejects', *Sunday Herald*, 17 December 1989, p. 3.
61 Lasker and Borg, p. 75.
62 Tom Tomlinson, 'Surrogate mothers and parental rights', *Hastings Center Report*, June 1984, p. 42.
63 Jo Wiles, 'The surrogate mother saga', *New Idea*, 26 March 1983, pp. 8, 9.
64 Dally.
65 Terese McFadden, 'Surrogate motherhood—refusing to relinquish a child', in Jocelynne A. Scutt (ed.), *The Baby Machine: Commercialisation of Motherhood*, McCulloch, Melbourne, 1988, p. 72.

66 Claire Lavoie, 'Husband runs off with surrogate mom!', *Weekly World News*, 26 May 1987.
67 Wiles, p. 9.
68 Vivien Harding, 'It just had to happen', *London Daily Mail*, 2 August 1984.
69 'Three in battle over custody', *West Australian*, 5 March 1991, p. 54.
70 Kate Inglis, *Living Mistakes: Mothers Who Consented To Adoption*, Allen & Unwin, Sydney, 1984, p. xi.
71 Gartland.
72 Corea, p. 231.
73 Robin Winkler and Margaret van Keppel, *Relinquishing Mothers in Adoption: Their Long-Term Adjustment*, Institute of Family Studies, Melbourne, 1984.
74 Reid, p. 5; Nicola Barry, 'When baby makes three illegal', *Guardian*, 11 December 1984, p. 10; Wiles, p. 9.
75 Elizabeth Kane, *Birth Mother*, Macmillan, Melbourne, 1990, p. 282.
76 Whitehead, in Klein, p. 142.
77 ibid., p. 140.
78 Patricia Foster, 'Women who experienced surrogacy speak out', in Klein p. 152.
79 Prudence Anderson, 'Caretaker mum', *Sun-Herald*, 22 September 1984.
80 'Baby not for sale', *Herald*, 1 August 1984, p. 3.
81 Harding.
82 Hyams, p. 10.
83 Dally, p. 11.
84 Grossman.
85 Kane, 1990 p. 272; Foster, in Klein, p. 153.
86 Whitehead, in Klein, pp. 142, 143.
87 Barrass, in Klein, p. 158.
88 Kane, 1988, p. 256 and epilogue.
89 Hyams, p. 10.
90 Foster, in Klein, p. 153.
91 Herbert T. Krimmel, 'The case against surrogate parenting', in Carol Levine (ed.), *Taking Sides: Clashing Views on Controversial Bio-Ethical Issues*, The Dushkin Publishing Group, Guildford, Connecticut, 1984, p. 54.
92 Peter Singer and Deane Wells, *The Reproduction Revolution: New Ways of Making Babies*, Oxford University Press, Oxford, 1984.
93 'Baby Sue', *Guardian*, 23 January 1985, p. 5.
94 Lori B. Andrews, 'Yours, mine and theirs', *Psychology Today*, December 1984, p. 24.
95 For a discussion of the consequences of AID, see Robyn Rowland, 'The social and psychological consequences of secrecy in artificial insemination by donor (AID) programmes', *Social Science in Medicine* 21, 4, 1985, pp. 391–6.

96 A. Clamar, 'Psychological implications of donor insemination', *American Journal of Psychoanalysis* 40, 1980.
97 S. Rubin, 'Letter to the editor', *School Paper CSU*, Northbridge, California, 1983.
98 Lasker and Borg, p. 153.
99 'Brain dead and pregnant: who will decide?', *Off Our Backs*, October 1986.
100 'Ruling by a court keeps a foetus alive', *Boston Globe*, 2 August 1986; 'Baby born to brain-dead woman dies', *Australian*, 18 August 1986.
101 Christopher Reed, 'Baby born to "dead" mother', *Age*, 1 August 1986; *Off Our Backs*, 1986; 'Special birthday', *Boston Globe*, 4 August 1987.
102 'Mother in a coma gives birth at 28 weeks', *Age*, 21 October 1986; 'Coma mother dies', *Age*, 23 October 1986.
103 Calvin Miller, 'Harvesting before the grim reaper', *Age*, 13 October 1986.
104 Calvin Miller, 'The brain-dead could be surrogates, say scientists', *Herald*, 24 June 1988, p. 1; Jackie Allender and Adam Courtenay, 'Surrogacy proposed for "dead" women', *Australian*, 25 June 1988.

5. THE VALUES OF MEDICAL SCIENCE

1 Ruth Bleier, *Science and Gender. A Critique of Biology and Its Theories on Women*, Pergamon Press, New York, 1984, p. 196.
2 Brian Easlea, *Science and Sexual Oppression—Patriarchy's Confrontation with Woman and Nature*, Weidenfeld & Nicolson, London, 1981, p. 7.
3 Ruth Hubbard, 'The Emperor doesn't wear any clothes: The impact of feminism on biology', in Dale Spender (ed.), *Men's Studies Modified. The impact of Feminism on the Academic Disciplines*, Pergamon Press, Oxford, 1981.
4 Emily Martin, *The Woman in the Body. A Cultural Analysis of Reproduction*, Beacon Press, Boston, 1987.
5 Barbara Ehrenreich and Deirdre English, *For Her Own Good: 150 Years of the Experts' Advice to Women*, Doubleday, New York, 1979, p. 17.
6 Bleier, pp. vii, 197.
7 Kathy Overfield, 'Dirty Fingers, Grime and Slag Heaps: Purity and the Scientific Ethic', in Spender, p. 241.
8 Libby Curran, 'Science Education: Did She Drop Out Or Was She Pushed?' in Lynda Birke, Wendy Faulkner, Sandy Best, Deidre Janson-Smith, Kathy Overfield (eds), *Alice Through The Microscope. The Power of Science Over Women's Lives*, Virago, London, 1980, pp. 40, 41.
9 Cited in Erik Arnold and Wendy Faulkner, 'Smothered by invention: the masculinity of technology', in Erik Arnold and Wendy Faulkner (eds), *Smothered By Invention, Technology in Women's Lives*, Pluto Press, London, 1985, p. 27.

10 Margaret Connor Versluysen, 'Midwives, medical men and "poor women labouring of child": lying-in hospitals in eighteenth-century London', in Helen Roberts (ed.), *Women, Health and Reproduction*, Routledge & Kegan Paul, London, 1981; Anna Hornbech Macgarvey, Women's Experiences of Medicalized Pregnancy and Childbirth, M.A. (Preliminary) Thesis, Deakin University, 1988; Ehrenreich and English.
11 Adrienne Rich, *Of Woman Born. Motherhood as Experience and Institution*, Virago, London, 1977.
12 Macgarvey, p. 17.
13 Macgarvey, Rich.
14 E. Willis, *Medical Dominance*, George Allen & Unwin, Sydney, 1983, p. 19.
15 Cited in Jo Murphy-Lawless, A Lexicon of the Female Body According to Obstetric Discourse, Third International Interdisciplinary Congress on Women, Dublin, July 1987, p. 7.
16 Philip McIntosh, 'Perth boost for test tube pregnancies', *West Australian*, 2 January 1988.
17 Judith N. Lasker and Susan Borg, *In Search of Parenthood. Coping with Infertility and High-Tech Conception*, Beacon Press, Boston, 1987, p. 60.
18 Martin, p. 151.
19 Margaret Pryke, Liselotte Muhlen and Kenneth Wade, 'Childbirth and Surgery: the experience of an Australian sample of 120 women during first birth', *New Doctor*, Autumn 1986, pp. 21–39; N.W. Cohen and L.J. Estner, *Silent Knife. Caesarean Prevention and Vaginal Birth After Caesarean*, Bergin & Gravey, South Hadley, Massachusetts, 1983; 'Private Doctors May Perform Cesarean Sections More Readily Than Their Hospital Counterparts', *Family Planning Perspectives*, January-February 1987, p. 26.
20 'Questions Routine Cesarean for Breech', *Ob.Gyn.News* 2, 6, 1987, p. 3.
21 Martin, p. 141.
22 Pryke et al., p. 21.
23 Joe Neel, 'Medico legal pressure, M.Ds' lack of patience cited in cesarean "epidemic"', *Ob.Gyn.News* 22, 10, 1987, p. 44.
24 Andrew Veitch, 'The Savage case over high tech babies', *Guardian*, 3 February 1986, p. 1.
25 J.R. Zorn, P. Boyer, A. Guichard, 'Never on a Sunday; Programming for IVF-ET and GIFT', *Lancet*, 14 February 1987, pp. 385–6; 'Fertility studies—overweight patients require more Pergonal for ovulation', *Ob.Gyn.News* 22, 12, 1987, p. 34; Peter Bromwich, Andrew Walker, Stephen Kennedy, Mary Wiley, David Little, Caroline Ross, Ian Sargent, Joan Bellinger, Helen O'Reilly, Andres Lopez-Bernal, Amy L. Brice, David Barlow, 'In vitro fertilisation in a small unit in the NHS', *British Medical Journal* 296, 1988, pp. 759–61.

26 Wendy Savage, *A Savage Enquiry. Who Controls Childbirth?* Virago, London, 1986, p. 175.
27 Pryke et al., p. 23.
28 Marion H. Hall, 'When a woman asks for a caesarean section', *British Medical Journal* 294, 24 January 1987, p. 201.
29 Neel, p. 44.
30 Martin, pp. 142, 144.
31 ibid., p. 20.
32 Ann Oakley. *The Captured Womb. A History of the Medical Care of Pregnant Women*, Blackwell, Oxford, 1984.
33 ibid., p. 281.
34 Ben Barker-Benfield, 'Sexual surgery in late-nineteenth-century America', *International Journal of Health Sciences* 5, 2, 1975, p. 285; Ehrenreich and English, p. 125; Easlea.
35 Isabel Wilkerson, 'Charges Against Doctor Bring Ire and Questions', *New York Times*, 11 December 1988; Gena Corea, *The Hidden Malpractice. How American Medicine Mistreats Women*, 2nd edition, Harper & Row, New York, 1985; Diana Scully, *Men Who Control Women's Health. The Miseducation of Obstetrician/Gynaecologists*, Houghton Mifflin, Boston, 1980.
36 Corea, p. 314.
37 Peter Benesh, 'Brainwashing and the CIA connection', Saturday Extra, *Age*, 12 March, 1988, p. 7.
38 Sandra Coney and Phillida Bunkle, 'An "unfortunate experiment" at National Women's', *Metro*, June 1987, p. 50. See also Sandra Coney, *The Unfortunate Experiment*, Penguin, Auckland, 1988.
39 ibid.
40 Coney and Bunkle, p. 50.
41 ibid., p. 56.
42 Andrew Pollack, 'Gene splicing payoff is near', Business Digest, *New York Times*, 10 June 1987, p. D1.
43 ibid., p. D6.
44 Marjorie Sun, 'Hot Market for Biotech Stocks in 1986', *Science* 233, 1 August 1986, pp. 516–17.
45 Sandra Atchison, 'Meet the Campus Capitalists of Bionic Valley, Science and Technology', *Business Week*, 5 May 1986, p. 114–15.
46 Sandra Blakeslee, 'Trying to make money making "test-tube" babies', *New York Times*, 17 May 1987, p. 6.
47 ibid., p. 6.
48 loc.cit.
49 Jenny Cullen, 'Why we are losing IVF researchers', *Australian*, 14 October 1986.
50 John Waugh, 'Breeding money', *Business Review Weekly*, 9 May 1986, p. 52.
51 'Embryo technique marketed in US', *Australian*, 16 May 1986.

52 'Road to sell is paved with good inventions; Innovation for sale', *Monash Review*, August 1986, p. 5.
53 Waugh, p. 59.
54 Susanna Rodell, 'IVF program goes private', *Herald*, 31 March 1988, p. 4.
55 Catherine Martin, 'A new and fertile field for investment', *Bulletin*, 24 June 1986.
56 ibid.
57 'Land of the raising son', *Sunday Press*, 12 February, 1989; Elisabeth Mealy, 'IVF baby lure for tourists', *Sun-Herald*, 24 July 1989.
58 Sandra Blakeslee, 1987.
59 ibid.
60 David Dickson, 'Universities and Industry: knowledge as commodity', *The New Politics of Science*, Pantheon, New York, 1984, pp. 56-106; Atchison, p. 115.
61 'Innovation for sale. Monash opens for business', *Monash Review*, August 1986, p. 5.
62 Sheldon Krimsky, 'Corporate academic ties in biotechnology. A report on research in progress', *Genewatch* 1, 5 and 6, 1984, pp. 3-4.
63 Andrew Veitch, 'Sugaring the pills', *Guardian*, 8 October 1986.
64 Pollack.
65 Tim Duncan, 'A happy marriage of business and microbiology', *Bulletin*, 6 May 1986.
66 'Dying for want of smear testing', *Age*, 16 December 1987; *FINRRAGE Newsletter*, May 1988, p. 5.
67 Rosemary West and Claire Miller, 'IVF investment questioned', *Age*, 12 May 1987, p. 3; 'No Conflict in IVF Interest: Fordham', *Age*, 15 May 1986; Mathew Ricketson, 'Cain backs joint $40m medical research venture', *Australian*, 22-23 November 1986; Peter Schumpeter, 'Why we are in debt to entrepreneurs', *Age*, 7 April 1986.
68 R.L. Martin, The University's Position, paper given at LES conference 27 March 1987, p. 5.
69 Philip McIntosh and David Broadbent, 'Kennan is reluctant to exempt universities', *Age*, 26 September 1985.
70 Mark Metherell, 'In vitro team ignored call for moratorium', *Age*, 4 June 1983, p. 16.
71 Michael Pirrie, 'New IVF Treatment stopped', *Age*, 2 April 1988, p. 1.
72 Mark Metherell, 'In vitro team ignored call for moratorium', *Age*, 4 June 1983, p. 16.
73 Charles Morgan, 'New Australian law on embryos still confuses researchers', *Nature* 325, 15 January 1987, p. 185; Carolyn Ford, 'Angry IVF doctors threaten to go abroad', *Weekend Australian*, 11 and 12 October 1986.

74 Jackie Allender, 'Legal delays force IVF scientists overseas', *Australian*, 15 April 1988.

75 Ann Westmore, 'The steps forward are not fast enough', *Age*, 9 March 1987.

76 J.L. Glick, 'Comments on papers by Dr Colman and Professor Linskens', in *Genetic Engineering: Commercial Opportunities in Australia*, Australian Government Publishing Service, Canberra, 1982.

77 ibid.

6. 'REPROSPEAK': THE LANGUAGE OF THE NEW REPRODUCTIVE TECHNOLOGIES

1 Robyn Rowland, 'Social implications of reproductive technology', *International Review of Natural Family Planning* 8, 3, 1984, pp. 189–205 (also published in Joseph N. Santamaria and Nicholas Tonti-Filippini (eds), *Proceedings of the 1984 Conference on Bioethics*, St Vincents Bioethics Centre, Melbourne, 1984, pp. 103–15.

2 See Chapter 4.

3 Robert M. Winston, 'Tubal microsurgery', in J. Studd (ed.), *Progress in Obstetrics and Gynaecology*, vol. 1, Churchill Livingston, Edinburgh, 1981.

4 'Conference de Gena Corea', in *Sortir La Maternité du Laboratoire*, Gouvernment du Quebec, Conseil du statut de la femme, 1988, p. 30.

5 *IVF and GIFT pregnancies Australia and New Zealand*, National Perinatal Statistics Unit, 1987, 1988, and 1990 for 1988.

6 Rosemary West, 'Victoria's first IVF surrogate mother may also be the last', *Age*, 20 April 1988.

7 Gena Corea and Susan Ince, 'Report of a survey of IVF Clinics in the US, in Patricia Spallone and Deborah Lynn Steinberg (eds), *Made to Order. The Myth of Reproductive and Genetic Progress*, Pergamon Press, Oxford, 1987, p. 141.

8 Judith N. Lasker and Susan Borg, *In Search of Parenthood, Coping with Infertility and High-Tech Conception*, Beacon Press, Boston, 1987, p. 57.

9 John C. McBain and Alan Trounson, 'Patient Management Treatment Cycle', in Carl Wood and Alan Trounson (eds), *Clinical in Vitro Fertilization*, Springer-Verlag, Berlin, 1984, p. 54; Robert Lee Hotz, 'Super-chilled embryos expected to spark a "scientific baby boom"', *Sydney Morning Herald*, 6 October 1986, p. 6.

10 Marge Piercy, *Circles in the Water. Selected Poems*, Alfred Knopf, New York, 1982, p. 263.

11 Christopher Joyce, 'Geneticists find the gene that determines sex', *New Scientist*, 24–31 December 1987, p. 29.

12 ibid., p. 29.

13 'Leading Fertility Centers Report Up to 40% In-Vitro Success Rates', *Ob.Gyn.News* 20, 5, 1985, p. 1.
14 M.F. Fathalla, 'Incessant Ovulation—A Factor in Ovarian Neoplasia?', *Lancet*, July 1971, p. 163.
15 Gabor T. Kovacs, Peter M. Dennis, Rhonda J. Shelton, Ken H. Outch, Robert A. McLean, David L. Healy and Henry G. Burger, 'Induction of ovulation with human pituitary gonadotrophin. Twelve years experience', *Medical Journal of Australia* 140, 10, 1984, p. 578.
16 Philip McIntosh, 'Pregnancy rate doubled in new IVF method', *Age*, 2 January 1988; Philip McIntosh, 'Perth boost for test tube pregnancies', *West Australian*, 2 January 1988; National Bioethics Consultative Committee, *Surrogacy*, draft report, 1988, 2.3.6.
17 Emily Martin, *The Woman in the Body. A cultural analysis of reproduction*, Beacon Press, Boston, 1987, p. 42.
18 Sue Downie, 'Fertility science goes back to nature', *Australian*, 25 April 1987.
19 ibid.
20 ibid.
21 Campbell Reid, 'Trade in human body parts sparks ethical debate', *Sunday Herald*, 15 July 1990, p. 15.
22 Annette Burfoot, 'Exploitation redefined: an interview with an IVF practitioner', *RFR/DFR* 18, 2, p. 29.
23 'Conference de Gena Corea', p. 31.
24 'Leading Fertility Centers Report…', p. 1.
25 Michael Pirrie, 'New IVF treatment stopped', *Age*, 2 April 1988.
26 'Baby craving: Science and Surrogacy', *Life Magazine*, June 1987.
27 Eve Glicksman, 'Miracle Moms', *Woman's World U.S.A.* 8 May 1990, p. 7; 'Increasing Costs, Other Problems Cited in Assisted Reproduction', *Ob.Gyn.News* 26, 1, 1991, p. 16; Claudine Escoffier-Lambiotte, 'The Fetal Medicine Debate. The Controversy over "Pre-birth Intervention"', *World Press Review*, 30 September 1983, p. 36.
28 National Bioethics Consultative Committee, 2.3.6; 2.6.3.
29 Nicholas Timmins, 'Why I am having a baby for my sister', *Times*, 23 September 1984, p. 11.
30 Nicola Barry, 'When baby makes three illegal', *Guardian*, 11 December 1984, p. 10.
31 Lucy Twomey, 'Surrogate Motherhood: a blessing or exploitation?', *Australian*, 2 May 1983.
32 Glenda Banks, 'I'm not playing God: IVF pioneer', *Sun*, 21 May 1987.
33 John A. Robertson, 'Surrogate mothers not so novel after all', in Carol Levine (ed.), *Taking Sides: Clashing Views on Controversial Bio-Ethical Issues*, Dushkin, Connecticut, 1984, p. 46.
34 '"Need to Know" on in vitro', *Sun*, 25 May 1984, p. 28.
35 Alan Trounson, 'In-Vitro Fertilisation—Past, Present and Future', *Search* 18, 3, 1987, p. 116.

36 Martin, p. 142.
37 'Male Factor Infertility Dx "Made Inappropriately" in 50% of Infertile', *Ob.Gyn.News* 22, 18, 1987; L. Poidevin, 'Social Implications of Pre-natal Cytogenetic Diagnosis', *Medical Journal of Australia* 143, 1985, p. 56.
38 Mark Ragg, 'The antenatal test with a big moral dilemma', *Australian*, 16 February 1988.
39 Deryn Thorpe, 'Contraceptive Vaccine on the Way', *Australian*, 13 October 1987. The concept of immunisation is an interesting one as it is used here and in other situations. In a discussion of the need to vaccinate children in India, Dr Banerjee talks critically of the World Health Organization's immunisation programme. He says that 'saturation spraying with vaccine' has been launched without epidemiological data. This is an interesting formulation, echoing as it does the language used of vermin and war enemies particularly during the Vietnam war and in Germany during World War II. Alone it stands as an interesting perception of children in the 'Third World'. ('Multi-million dollar vaccination drive against infant mortality', *Nature* 325, 29 January 1987.)
40 Rosemary West, 'Feminist urges women to boycott new IVF study', *Age*, 17 May 1986, p. 18.
41 Susan Downie, 'Help on way for infertile males', *Australian*, 17 December 1986 and 'Fertility science goes back to nature', *Australian*, 25 April 1987.
42 'Baby Craving: Science and Surrogacy', in *Life Magazine*, June 1987, p. 25.
43 Lasker and Borg, p. 98.
44 ibid., p. 118.
45 'Orphaned embryos may be left to thaw', *Sydney Morning Herald*, 4 September 1984; 'Scientists fear embryo trade', *Age*, 6 October 1987; Andrew Veitch, 'More frozen embryos wait to find mothers', *Guardian*, 17 July 1984.
46 Ronald Smothers, 'Tennessee Judge Awards Custody of 7 Frozen Embryos to Woman', *New York Times National*, 22 September 1989.
47 'Grading scale helps assess embryo quality in in vitro fertilization', *Ob.Gyn.News* 21, 2, 1986, p. 39; 'Low IVF pregnancy rate tied to "wayward embryos"', *Ob.Gyn.News* 21, 20, 1986, p. 18.
48 Ragg.
49 Downie, 1986.
50 Lasker and Borg, p. 93.
51 ibid., p. 101.
52 Michael R. Harrison, 'Unborn: Historical perspective of the fetus as a patient', *Pharos*, Winter 1982, pp. 19, 22.
53 'Technology for Improving Fetal Therapy Advancing Exponentially', *Ob.Gyn.News* 22, 12, 1987, p. 31.

54 Bill Hitchings, ' "New baby" needs nurturing, caution proud doctors', *Herald*, 8 April 1985, p. 4.
55 Ruth Gledhill, 'He's Daddy of Them All!' Tempo Talk, *Sydney Morning Herald*; Catherine Martin, 'A new and fertile field for investment', *Bulletin*, 24 June 1986; Susan Downie, 'Fathers of IVF push the barriers further', *Australian*, 17 November 1986.
56 Christopher Hanson, 'Baby farming: the modern moral dilemma', *Australian*, 26 November 1987.
57 'IVF Team in Share issue bid', *Sun*, 28 June 1986.
58 'Trying to make money making "Test-Tube" babies', *New York Times*, 17 May 1987, p. 6.
59 Catherine Martin; Tim Duncan, 'A Happy Marriage of Business and Micro Biology', *Bulletin*, 6 May 1986.
60 'Low IVF pregnancy rate...', p. 18; Twomey.
61 'Baby Craving', p. 7.
62 Escoffier-Lambiotte, p. 36.
63 'Baby Craving', p. 7.
64 Gena Corea, *The Mother Machine: From Artificial Insemination to Artificial Wombs*, Harper & Row, New York, 1985.
65 Glennys Bell, 'Our Awesome future—the brave new bio-tech world', *Bulletin*, 6 May 1986.
66 Cited in Lasker and Borg, p. 124.

7. MOTHERHOOD AND INFERTILITY: MEDICAL SCIENCE CO-OPTS IDEOLOGY AND DESIRE

1 Adrienne Rich, *Of Woman Born: Motherhood as Experience and Institution*, Virago, London, 1977, p. 279.
2 Janice Raymond, 'The spermatic market: surrogate stock and liquid assets', in *Reproductive and Genetic Engineering. Journal of International Feminist Analysis*, 1, 1, 1988, p. 70.
3 Effective contraception in the last twenty to sixty years has given women more choice as to how many children they would have and when they would have them. Ironically, contraception may have taken away that choice for many women. For example, the pill may switch off the hypothalamus, stopping ovulation and production of eggs; an infection from using an IUD may lead to pelvic inflammatory disease which leads to infertility.
4 Barbara Sichtermann, *Femininity. The Politics of the Personal*, ed. Helga Geyer-Ryan, translated by John Whitlam, Polity Press, Oxford, 1983, pp. 18, 19.
5 Leta S. Hollingworth, 'Social devices for impelling women to bear and rear children', *American Journal of Sociology*, 22, 1916, p. 25.
6 ibid., p. 29.
7 Ben Wattenberg, 'The birth dearth' (excerpt), *U.S. News and World Report*, June 22 1987, pp. 56–65.

8 J.M. Bardwick, 'Evolution and parenting', *Journal of Social Issues* 30, 1974, pp. 39, 38; J.M. Bardwick *In Transition*, Holt, Rinehart & Winston, New York, 1979, p. 79.

9 Douglas C. Kimmell, *Adulthood and Aging*, John Wiley & Sons, New York, 1980, p. 166.

10 Jeffner Allen, 'Motherhood: the annihilation of women', and Joyce Trebilcot (ed.), in *Mothering: Essays in Feminist Theory*, Rowman Allenheld, New Jersey, 1984, p. 318.

11 Stephanie Dowrick and Sybil Grundberg (eds), *Why Children?* Penguin, Melbourne, 1980, p. 7.

12 Bronwyn Davies and D'anne Welch, 'Motherhood and feminism: are they compatible? The ambivalence of mothering', *Australian and New Zealand Journal of Sociology* 22, 1986, pp. 419, 424.

13 Jessie Bernard, *The Future of Marriage*, Bantam Books, New York, 1973.

14 Nancy Chodorow, *The Reproduction of Mothering: Psychoanalysis and The Sociology of Gender*, University of California Press, Los Angeles, 1978, p. 31.

15 Dowrick and Grundberg, p. 7.

16 Adrienne Rich, *On Lies, Secrets and Silence*, Virago, London, 1980, p. 260.

17 Rich, 1976, p. 13.

18 Sarah Ruddick, 'Maternal thinking', in Trebilcot, p. 220.

19 ibid., p. 221.

20 Raymond, p. 73.

21 Irena Klepfisz, in Dowrick and Grundberg, p. 18.

22 Barbara Wishart, 'Motherhood within patriarchy—a radical feminist perspective', in *All Her Labours: Embroidering The Framework*, Hale & Iremonger, Sydney, 1984, p. 96.

23 L.G. Calhoun and J.W. Selby, 'Voluntary childlessness, involuntary childlessness and having children: A study of social perceptions', *Family Relations* 29, 1980, pp. 181-83; See also E. Peck and J. Sanderowitz, *Pronatalism: The Myth of Mom and Apple Pie*, Thomas Y. Crowell & Co., New York, 1974; P.H. Jamison, L.R. Franzini and R.M. Kaplan, 'Some assumed characteristics of voluntarily childfree men and women', *Psychology of Women Quarterly* 4, 1979, pp. 266-73; Jean E. Veevers, *Childless by Choice*, Butterworth, Toronto, 1980; Robyn Rowland, 'An exploratory study of the child-free lifestyle', in *Australian and New Zealand Journal of Sociology* 18, 1, 1982, pp. 17-30.

24 Personal communication, first published in Robyn Rowland, *Woman Herself: A Transdisciplinary Perspective on Women's Identity*, Oxford University Press, Melbourne, 1988; Veevers; Rowland, 1982.

25 M. Movius, 'Voluntary childlessness—the ultimate liberation', *Family Co-ordinators* 25, 1976, pp. 57-63.

26 Cited in Eileen Alderton, 'What the latest research means to childless couples', *Australian Women's Weekly* 28 July 1982, p. 65.

27 M.G.R. Hull, D.N. Joyce, F.N. McLeod and B.D. Ray, 'Human in vitro fertilization, in vivo sperm penetration of cervical mucus, and unexplained infertility', *Lancet*, 4 August 1984, pp. 245-6.

28 Naomi Pfeffer and Anne Woollett, *The Experience of Infertility*, Virago, London, 1983. The Office of Technology Assessment in America found that between 1965 and 1982 'The percentage of couples infertile has changed only slightly, rising from 13.3% to 13.9%' (p. 51, OTA Report, *Infertility*). There are few studies which accurately assess the rates of infertility as opposed to increasing decisions by couples to live without children. For example, Johnson and her colleagues point out that there are no published British data on the prevalence of what she calls voluntary infertility. In their study of the medical records of women born in 1950 and in 1935, on the lists of ten practices in England, Johnson et al. found that although there was a significant increase in voluntary childlessness between the group of women born in 1935 and those born in 1950 (3.2% to 11%) there was no evidence of increased involuntary childlessness in these two age groups. Figures for the group in 1950 indicated a 3.3% rate of involuntary childlessness compared to a 4.5% rate for the women born in 1935. (Gina Johnson, et al., 'Infertile or Childless by Choice? A Multipractice survey of women aged 35 and 50', *British Medical Journal* 294, 1987, p. 806.

29 William R. Keye, 'Strategy for avoiding iatrogenic infertility', *Contemporary Obstetrics and Gynaecology* 19, 1982, pp. 185-95.

30 'Earlier more liberal use of laparoscopy is advised', *Ob.Gyn.News* 19, 24, 1984.

31 'Find IUD use increases infertility risk in nulliparous', *Ob.Gyn.News* 20, 10 1985; Connie Levitt, '$15m for IUD victims denounced', *Sydney Morning Herald*, 5 June 1987; 'Preserving fertility a therapy concern even in young', *Ob.Gyn.News* 21, 13, 1986, p. 2; 'Internists "often poor" at diagnosing, treating PID', *Ob.Gyn. News* 22, 10, 1987, pp. 3, 29; 'Early ovarian failure tied to prior abdominal surgery', *Ob.Gyn.News* 22, 1, 1987, p. 2.

32 V. Baukloh, H.G. Bohnet, M. Trapp, W. Feichtinger and P. Kemeter, 'Biocides in human follicular fluid' (abstr.), *Journal of in Vitro Fertilization and Embryo Transfer* 1, 2, 1984, p. 98; Michael Odenwald, 'Environmental toxins are blamed for increase in human infertility', *German Tribune* 1362, 1989, p. 13. There is increasing concern about the effect of environmental and industrial pollution on egg and sperm quality. A number of articles have appeared emphasising that male fertility may be declining because of pollution. Chemicals and PCBs have been found in semen samples within America.

33 Renate Klein, *The Exploitation of a Desire: Women's Experiences With in Vitro Fertilisation*, Deakin University Press, Geelong, 1989, p. 10.
34 Barbara Burton, The need for reproductive control and self-determination for infertile women, Paper presented to Liberation or Loss? conference, Canberra, May, 1986.
35 Klein.
36 Christine Crowe, 'Women want it: in-vitro fertilization and women's motives for participation', *Women's Studies International Forum* 8, 6, 1985 p. 550; Miriam Mazor, 'Barren couples', *Psychology Today* 12, 1979, pp. 101-12; Ann Atkin, quoted in Joanne Anderson, 'Women who know what it means to be infertile', *Sun Living Supplement*, 17 March 1987, p. 2.
37 See for example: 'Exercise, stress and infertility', *New Scientist*, 8 November 1984, p. 19; Be Bonham, 'Men's fertility threatened by environment', *Sydney Morning Herald*, 9 November 1986.
38 Paul Entwhistle, quoted in Denise Winn, 'The fertile mind', *New Idea*, 6 August 1988, p. 29.
39 Personal communication from Geraldine Stevens, on her studies with infertile women.
40 Alison Solomon, 'Sometimes Pergonal kills', in Klein, pp. 41-50.
41 Cited in Deborah Smith, 'Fighting infertility', *National Times*, 19 October 1984, pp. 25-7.
42 Diane Houghton and Peter Houghton, *Coping With Childlessness*, George Allen & Unwin, London, 1984, pp. 144, 145.
43 Rich, 1977, p. 253.
44 Chodorow, p. 7.
45 Rich, 1977, p. 279.
46 ibid., p. 280.
47 Janice Raymond, 'Making international connections: surrogacy, the traffic in women and demythologizing motherhood', in *Sortir La Maternité du Laboratoire*, Gouvernement du Quebec, Conseil du Statut de la Femme, 1988, pp. 362-3.
48 Judith N. Lasker and Susan Borg, *In Search of Parenthood: Coping With Infertility and High-Tech Conception*, Beacon Press, Boston, 1987, p. 16.
49 ibid., p. 16; my own research with AID couples supports this.
50 Barbara Katz Rothman, 'How science is redefining parenting', *Ms*, July-August 1982, pp. 154-8.
51 Raymond, p. 70.
52 Jo Sutton and Scarlet Friedman, 'Fatherhood: bringing it all back home', in Scarlet Friedman and Elizabeth Sarah (eds), *On The Problems of Men: Two Feminist Conferences*, The Women's Press, London, 1982, p. 124.
53 Scarlet Pollock and Jo Sutton, 'Father's rights, woman's losses', *Women's Studies International Forum* 8, 6, 1985, pp. 593-600.

54 Glenn Martin, letter to *National Times*, 20-26 May 1983, p. 44.
55 Barbara Hutton, 'Dividing the cost of child support', *Age*, 31 October 1986, p. 22.
56 Phyllis Chesler, *Mothers On Trial: The Battle For Children And Custody*, The Seal Press, Washington, 1986.
57 Carol Smart, ' "There is of course the distinction dictated by nature": law and the problem of paternity', in Michelle Stanworth (ed.), *Reproductive Technologies: Gender, Motherhood and Medicine*, Polity Press, Cambridge, 1987, pp. 111-12, 116.
58 Pollock and Sutton, p. 599.
59 Raymond, p. 67.
60 'Agony of a father denied any say in the fate of his baby', *Australian*, 3 March 1987; Clare Dyer, 1987, 'Father fails in attempt to stop girlfriend's abortion', *British Medical Journal* 294, 1987, pp. 631-2.

8. RIGHTS, RESPONSIBILITIES AND RESISTANCE

1 Chet Fleming, 'If We Can Keep A Severed Head Alive ...', *British Medical Journal* 297, 1988, p. 1048.
2 I prefer to use the term 'users' of reproductive technology rather than 'consumers'; in reality all members of our society are consumers of this technology in one form or another and it affects all of us equally in the long term.
3 Carole Pateman, *The Sexual Contract*, Polity Press, Cambridge, 1988.
4 Beverley Wildung Harrison, *Our Right To Choose. Toward A New Ethic of Abortion*, Beacon Press, Boston, 1983, pp. 197-8.
5 Carole Pateman, pp. 14-15.
6 Catharine A. MacKinnon, *Feminism Unmodified. Discourses On Life and Law*, Harvard University Press, Cambridge, Massachusetts, 1987, p. 16.
7 Harrison, p. 197 (my emphasis).
8 Rosalind Pollack Petchesky, *Abortion and Woman's Choice. The State, Sexuality, and Reproductive Freedom*, Longman, New York, 1984, p. 395.
9 Susan Sherwin, 'A Feminist Approach to Ethics', *Resources for Feminist Research (RFR/DRF)* 16, 3, 1987, pp. 25-8.
10 Max Charlesworth, 'Reasons For and Against Surrogate Motherhood', in Marie Meggitt (ed.), *Surrogacy—In Whose Interest?* Proceedings of the National Conference Melbourne, February 1991, Mission of St James and St John, Melbourne, 1991, p. 61.
11 Petchesky.
12 Robin Morgan, *The Anatomy of Freedom. Feminism, Physics and Global Politics*, Martin Robertson, Oxford, 1982, p. 4.
13 Bell Hooks, *Feminist Theory: From Margin To Center*, South End Press, Boston, 1984, pp. 5-6.

14 R. Hull, 'Informed Consent: Patient's Right or Patient's Duty', *Journal of Medicine and Philosophy* 10, 2, 1985, pp. 183-97; F.J. Ingelfinger, 'Informed (but uneducated) Consent', *New England Journal of Medicine* 287, 9, 1972, pp. 465-6.
15 Gena Corea, *The Mother Machine: Reproductive Technologies from Artificial Insemination to Artificial Wombs*, Harper & Row, New York, 1985.
16 ibid.
17 *Ob.Gyn.News* 21, 10, 1986, pp. 15-31, p. 36a.
18 Janice Raymond, 'Informed Consent and Transsexual Surgery', *Medicine Science and the Law: Informed Consent*, Symposia 1986, Law Reform Commission of Victoria, Melbourne, p. 44.
19 Barbara Katz Rothman, *The Tentative Pregnancy. Prenatal Diagnosis and the Future of Motherhood*, Penguin, New York, 1987, p. 51.
20 Gena Corea, p. 227.
21 Barbara Katz Rothman, p. 243.
22 Susan Himmelweit, 'More Than A Woman's Right to Choose?', *Feminist Review* 29, 1988, p. 50.
23 ibid., p. 43.
24 Jane McLoughlin, 'Playing Russian roulette with employees', *Guardian*, 10 July 1986.
25 Barbara Katz Rothman, 'The meanings of choice in reproductive technology', in Rita Arditti, Renate Duelli Klein and Shelley Minden (eds), *Test-Tube Women. What future for motherhood?*, Pandora Press, London, 1984, p. 30.
26 Christine Ewing and Renate Klein, 'Joint Resistance: Women Oppose the Technological Take-over of Life', *Reproductive and Genetic Engineering. Journal of International Feminist Analysis* 2, 3, 1989, pp. 279-284.
27 Gail Vines, 'Transplanted eggs can create ovaries', *New Scientist*, 10 February 1990, p. 12.
28 Carlo Bulletti et al., 'Extracorporeal Perfusion of the Human Uterus', *American Journal of Obstetrics and Gynaecology* 154, 3, 1986, pp. 683-688; Carlo Bulletti et al., 'Early Human Pregnancy in vitro utilising an artificially perfused uterus', *Fertility and Sterility* 49, 6, 1988, p. 991-6.
29 Rosalind Herlands, 'Biological manipulation for producing and nurturing mammalian embryos', *The Custom-Made Child? Woman Centered Perspectives*, The Humana Press, New Jersey, 1981.
30 John Buuck, 'Ethics of reproductive engineering', *Perspectives* 3, 9, 1987, pp. 545-7.
31 Edward Grossman, 'The obsolescent mother: A Scenario', *Atlantic* 227, 1971, pp. 39-50.
32 Dick Teresi and Kathleen McAuliffe, 'Male Pregnancy', *Omni*, December 1985, pp. 51-118.

33 'Outrage over male pregnancy move', *Sunday Mail* (Adelaide), 27 November 1988, p. 59.
34 Robin Kent, 'The birth of the male mother', *Weekend Australian*, 17-18 May 1986, p. 15.
35 Teresi and McAuliffe, 'Male Pregnancy'; also Nicole Silverman, 'Transsexuals yearn for motherhood', *Telegraph*, 17 May 1986; 'Transsexuals see IVF program as their chance to become mothers', *Sydney Morning Herald*, 5 July 1984; 'Babies for men possible in two years', *Herald*, 21 November 1988.
36 Teresi and McAuliffe, p. 118.
37 'Transsexuals see IVF program as their chance ...'.
38 'The man who became a woman', *New Idea*, 22 March 1986, pp. 8-9.
39 ibid., my emphasis.
40 Janice Raymond, *The Transsexual Empire. The Making of the She-Male*, Beacon Press, Boston, 1979.
41 Laurence Karp, *Genetic Engineering: Threat or Promise?*, Prentice-Hall, Chicago, 1976, p. 162.
42 Lynda Lange, 'Feminism and political choice: Reproductive labour and the tension between collectivism, cultural nationalism, and individualism', *Resources for Feminist Research (RFR/DRF)* 16, 3, 1987, pp. 38-41.
43 Kate Millett, *The Prostitution Papers*, Avon Books, New York, 1973, p. 96.
44 D. Wrong, *Power: Its Forms, Bases and Uses*, Basil Blackwell, Oxford, 1979, p. 111.
45 Andrea Dworkin, *Right Wing Women: The Politics of Domesticated Females*, The Women's Press, London, 1978, p. 234.
46 Frances Evans, 'Managers and labourers: women's attitudes to reproductive technology', in Wendy Faulkner and Erik Arnold *Smothered By Invention: Technology in Women's Lives*, Pluto Press, London, 1985, p. 120.
47 Catherine Kohler-Riessman, 'Women and medicalisation: a new perspective', *Social Policy* 14, 1, 1983, pp. 3-18.
48 Quoted in Peter Singer and Deane Wells, *The Reproduction Revolution: New Ways of Making Babies*, Oxford University Press, Oxford, 1984, p. 22.
49 Judith N. Lasker and Susan Borg, *In Search of Parenthood: Coping With Infertility and High-Tech Conception*, Beacon Press, Boston, 1987, p. 30.
50 Dworkin, p. 183.
51 Pateman, p. 193.
52 Examples of these publications include Rita Arditti, Renate D. Klein, Shelley Minden (eds), *Test Tube Women: What Future For Motherhood; Man-Made Women: How New Reproductive Technologies Affect Women*, Hutchinson, London, 1985; Patricia Spallone and

Deborah Lynn Steinberg *Made To Order: The Myth of Reproductive and Genetic Progress*, Pergamon, Oxford, 1987. A further example is the development of the prestigious journal *Issues in Reproductive and Genetic Engineering: Journal of International Feminist Analysis.*

53. Further examples include the appearance of FINRRAGE members Robyn Rowland, Ditta Bartels, Lariane Fonseca, Heather Dietrich and others from the network as witnesses before various government committees including the Waller Committee in Victoria, the Cornwall Committee in South Australia, the Law Reform Commission in New South Wales and Victoria, and the Federal Senate's Select Committee on the Human Embryo Experimentation Bill.

54 Dworkin, 1978, p. 52.

55 Dworkin, 1978, p. 53.

INDEX

Robyn Rowland, a social psychologist and Associate Professor in women's studies at Deakin University, has addressed meetings of M.P.s and state government committees in England, Ireland, the United States, and Australia. She has published widely on reproductive technology and is a contributor to many books in this area, including *Test-tube Women: What Future for Motherhood?* and *Man-made Women: How New Reproductive Technologies Affect Women*. She is the author of *Woman Herself: A Transdisciplinary Perspective on Women's Identity*.

